TABLE OF CONTENTS

1 INTRODUCTION

Crohn's disease is one of a group of diseases known as inflammatory bowel disease (IBD). Ulcerative colitis is another type of IBD.

Crohn's disease is an autoimmune-mediated inflammatory condition. This means the immune system mistakenly attacks the body's own cells, thinking they are harmful when they are not.

Crohn's can affect any part of the gastrointestinal (GI) tract, from the mouth to the anus. Symptoms mainly involve the intestinal system, but they can also affect the skin, joints, bones, eyes, kidneys, and liver.

There are many theories about why Crohn's develops, including genetic factors, problems with the gut microbiome, and environmental exposure.

One prominent theory is that it is an autoimmune condition. This means that the immune system mistakenly attacks healthy cells in the body. As the immune system interacts with different organisms, this may trigger inflammation and intestinal damage.

In someone with Crohn's disease, bacteria in the digestive tract may trigger an immune response that continues to occur, resulting in ongoing intestinal damage.

There are five types of Crohn's disease, according to the Crohn's and Colitis Foundation.

They are:

- Ileocolitis: The most common type, this affects the end of the small intestine and the large intestine, or colon.

- Ileitis: The only affects the ileum, or small intestine.

- Gastroduodenal Crohn's disease: This affects the stomach and the duodenum, which is the beginning of the small intestine.

- Jejunoileitis: This causes patches of inflammation in the jejunum, the upper part of the small intestine.

- Crohn's (granulomatous) colitis: This affects only the colon.

Symptoms range from vomiting to rectal bleeding and depend to some extent on the type.

2 WHAT IS CROHN'S DISEASE?

Crohn's disease is a long-term condition that causes inflammation of the lining of the digestive system.

Inflammation can affect any part of the digestive system, from the mouth to the back passage, but most commonly occurs in the last section of the small intestine (ileum) or the large intestine (colon).

Common symptoms can include:

- diarrhoea
- abdominal pain
- fatigue (extreme tiredness)
- unintended weight loss
- blood and mucus in your faeces (stools)

People with Crohn's disease sometimes go for long periods without symptoms, or with very mild symptoms. This is known as remission. Remission can be followed by periods where symptoms flare up and become particularly troublesome.

Why it happens

The exact cause of Crohn's disease is unknown. However, research suggests that a combination of factors may be responsible. These include:

- genetics - genes that you inherit from your parents may increase your risk of developing Crohn's disease
- the immune system - the inflammation may be caused by a problem with the immune system (the body's defence against infection

and illness) that causes it to attack healthy bacteria in the gut

- previous infection - a previous infection may trigger an abnormal response from the immune system
- smoking - smokers with Crohn's disease usually have more severe symptoms than non-smokers
- environmental factors - Crohn's disease is most common in westernised countries, such as the UK, and least common in poorer parts of the world, such as Africa, which suggests the environment (particularly sanitation) has a part to play

2.1   CAUSES OF CROHN'S DISEASE

The exact cause of Crohn's disease is unknown. Most researchers think that it is caused by a combination of factors.

These are thought to be:

- genetics
- the immune system
- smoking
- previous infection
- environmental factors

There is no evidence to suggest a particular diet can cause Crohn's disease, although changes to your diet can be helpful to control certain symptoms and maybe recommended by your specialist or dietitian.

Genetics

There is evidence to suggest that genetics plays a role in the development of Crohn's disease.

Researchers have identified over 200 different genes that are more common in people with Crohn's disease than in the general population.

There is also evidence that Crohn's disease can run in families. About 3 in 20 people with the condition have a close relative (mother, father, sister or brother) who also has Crohn's disease. If you have an identical twin with Crohn's disease, you have a 70% chance of also developing it.

The fact that Crohn's disease is more common in some ethnic groups than in others also suggests that genetics plays an important role.

The immune system

The immune system provides protection against harmful bacteria that could potentially find their way into the digestive system.

The digestive system is also home to many different types of so-called "friendly bacteria" that help to digest food. The immune system usually recognises these bacteria and lets them do their job without attacking them.

However, in Crohn's disease, it seems that something disrupts the immune system, which sends a special protein, known as tumour necrosis factor alpha (TNF-alpha), to kill all bacteria, regardless of whether they are friendly or not. This causes most of the inflammation associated with Crohn's disease.

Previous infection

In certain genetically susceptible individuals, a previous childhood infection may lead to an abnormal immune response, causing the symptoms of Crohn's disease.

One possible source of this infection is a bacterium called Mycobacterium avium subspecies paratuberculosis (MAP). MAP is commonly found in cows, sheep and goats.

Research has found that people with Crohn's disease are seven times more likely to have traces of MAP in their blood compared with the general population.

MAP has been known to survive the pasteurisation process (where milk is treated with heat to kill bacteria), so it is possible that people have become infected with MAP by drinking milk from contaminated animals.

However, the exact role that MAP may play in the development of Crohn's disease is uncertain and some researchers dispute this theory.

Smoking

Aside from family history and ethnic background, smoking is the most important risk factor for Crohn's disease. Smokers are twice as likely to develop Crohn's disease compared with non-smokers.

Furthermore, people with Crohn's disease who smoke usually experience more severe symptoms compared with those with the condition who do not smoke.

Environmental factors

There are two unusual aspects of Crohn's disease that have led many researchers to believe that environmental factors may play a part. These are explained below.

Crohn's disease is a "disease of the rich". The highest number of cases occurs in developed parts of the world, such as the UK and US, and the lowest number in developing parts of the world, such as Africa and Asia.

Crohn's disease became much more widespread from the 1950s onwards.

This suggests that there is something associated with modern, western lifestyles that increases a person's risk of developing Crohn's disease.

One theory to explain this is known as the hygiene hypothesis. It suggests that as children grow up in increasingly germ-free environments, their immune system does not fully develop due to a lack of exposure to childhood infections. However, there is little in the way of hard, scientific evidence to support this theory.

An alternative theory is the cold-chain hypothesis, which suggests that the increase in the number of cases of Crohn's disease might be linked to the increased use of refrigerators after the Second World War.

2.2   Symptoms of Crohn's disease

The symptoms of Crohn's vary depending on which part of the digestive system is inflamed.

Common symptoms include:

- recurring diarrhoea
- abdominal pain and cramping, which is usually worse after eating
- extreme tiredness (fatigue)
- unintended weight loss
- blood and mucus in your faeces (stools)

You may find that you experience all or only one of the above. Some people experience severe symptoms, but others only have mild problems.

There may be long periods that last for weeks or months where you have very mild or no symptoms (known as remission), followed by periods where the symptoms are particularly troublesome (known as flare ups or relapses).

Less common symptoms include:

- high temperature (fever) of 38°C (100°F) or above
- feeling sick (nausea)
- being sick (vomiting)
- joint pain and swelling (arthritis)
- inflammation and irritation of the eyes (uveitis)
- areas of painful, red and swollen skin - most often of the legs
- mouth ulcers

Children with Crohn's disease may grow at a slower rate than expected because the inflammation can prevent the body absorbing nutrients from food.

When to seek medical advice

You should contact your doctor if you have:

- persistent diarrhoea
- persistent abdominal pain
- unexplained weight loss
- blood in your faeces (stools)

You should also see your doctor if you are concerned about your child's development.

2.3 DIAGNOSING CROHN'S DISEASE

A number of different tests may be needed to diagnose Crohn's disease, as it has similar symptoms to several other conditions.

Initial assessment

During your initial assessment, it is likely that your doctor will ask you about the pattern of your symptoms and check whether there may be any contributing causes, such as:

- diet

- recent travel - for example, you may have developed travellers' diarrhoea while travelling abroad

- whether you are taking any medication, including any over-the-counter (OTC) medicines

- whether you have a family history of Crohn's disease

Your doctor may also carry out a series of standard tests to assess your general state of health. For example, they may:

- check your pulse
- check your blood pressure
- measure your weight and height
- measure your temperature
- examine your abdomen (tummy)

Blood tests

Your doctor may then arrange a series of blood tests. These can be used to assess:

- the levels of inflammation in your body
- whether you have an infection

- whether you are anaemic (have low levels of red blood cells), which could suggest you are malnourished

Stool sample

You may be asked to provide a stool sample that can be checked for blood and mucus. It can also be used to determine whether your symptoms are being caused by a parasitic infection such as roundworm, or other infections.

After you have provided a stool and blood sample, you will probably be referred a gastroenterologist (a specialist in conditions of the digestive system) who can discuss the results with you and can carry out the tests described below if they are necessary.

Colonoscopy

A colonoscopy is a test used to examine the inside of your colon. It involves inserting a long flexible tube, known as an endoscope, into your colon through your back passage (rectum).

The endoscope has a light and a camera on the end. The camera can be used to send images to a television screen. These will show the level and extent of inflammation inside your colon.

The endoscope can also be fitted with surgical tools that can be used to take a number of small tissue samples from different sections of your digestive system. This is known as a biopsy. The procedure may feel uncomfortable but it is not painful.

These tissue samples will be examined under a microscope for the cell changes known to occur in cases of Crohn's disease.

Wireless capsule endoscopy

A wireless capsule endoscopy is a new type of test that involves swallowing a small capsule (about the size of a large vitamin tablet). The capsule works its way down to your small intestines where it transmits images to a recording device worn on a belt or in a small shoulder bag.

A few days after the test, the capsule passes out of your body in a stool. The capsule is disposable so you do not have to worry about retrieving it from your stools.

As this is a relatively new test, availability may be limited. In some cases, scans called MRE or CTE may be used instead of a capsule endoscopy.

MRE and CTE scans

Scans called magnetic resonance enterography/enteroclysis (MRE) or computerised tomography enterography/enteroclysis (CTE) may be used to examine the small intestine in people with suspected Crohn's disease.

Before having these scans you will either need to drink a harmless liquid called a contrast agent (enterography), or a contrast agent may be placed through a tube in your nose that leads to your small intestine (enteroclysis). These contrast agents allow your small intestine to show up more clearly during the scans.

During an MRE scan, magnetic fields and radio waves are used to produce detailed images of your small intestines. During CTE scans, several X-rays are taken and assembled by computer to create a detailed image.

These tests are increasingly used instead of a small bowel enema or small bowel follow-through because they allow more detailed examination of the small intestine and MRE scans also avoid any exposure to X-ray radiation.

Small bowel enema or small bowel follow-through

A small bowel enema (SBE) and small bowel follow through (SBFT) are two similar tests that have traditionally been used to examine the whole of the inside of the small intestine, usually at the point where it meets the colon. Thay are sometimes used because only about the last 20 cm is usually seen during colonoscopy.

During an SBE/SBFT, a local anaesthetic spray is used to numb the inside of your nose and throat. A tube is passed down your nose and into your throat, before being threaded into your small intestines. This can feel unpleasant at first, but most people find that they get used to the sensation after a few minutes.

A harmless liquid called barium is passed down the tube. The barium coats the lining of your small intestines so that they show up clearly on X-rays. A series of X-ray images will then be taken. The images can often highlight the areas of narrowing and inflammation that are caused by Crohn's disease.

After the test, you will be advised to drink plenty of fluid to help wash the barium out of your body. You may notice that your stools look white for the first few days after having an SBE/SBFT. This is perfectly normal and it is nothing to worry about.

2.4 TREATMENT FOR CROHN'S DISEASE

There is currently no cure for Crohn's disease, but treatment can help improve the symptoms.

The main aims of treatment are to:

- reduce symptoms - known as inducing remission (remission is a period without symptoms)
- maintain remission

In children, treatment also aims to promote healthy growth and development.

Your treatment will usually be provided by a range of healthcare professionals, including specialist doctors (such as gastroenterologists or surgeons), doctors and specialist nurses.

Reducing symptoms

If you have Crohn's disease and it's causing moderate or severe symptoms, this is known as "active disease". Treatment for active Crohn's disease usually involves medication, but surgery is sometimes the best option.

Initial treatment

In most cases, the first treatment offered is steroid medication (corticosteroids) to reduce the inflammation. Examples of corticosteroids used for Crohn's disease include prednisolone tablets or hydrocortisone injections.

These medications are often effective in reducing the symptoms of Crohn's disease, but they can have significant side effects - such as:

- weight gain

- swelling of the face

- increased vulnerability to infections

- thinning and weakening of the bones (osteopenia and osteoporosis)

Due to these possible side effects, your dose will be gradually reduced when your symptoms start to improve.

If you prefer, you may be able to choose to have a milder steroid called budesonide, or a type of medication called a 5-aminosalicylate (such as mesalazine), as an alternative initial treatment. These medications have fewer side effects, but they are less effective.

In children or young people where there are concerns about growth and development, a special liquid diet may be recommended as an initial treatment. This is known as an elemental or polymeric diet and it can help to reduce inflammation by allowing your digestive system to recover, while ensuring that they get all the nutrients they need.

Additional treatment

If your symptoms flare up twice or more during 12 months, or if your symptoms return when your steroid dose is reduced, further treatment may be necessary.

In these cases, medicines to suppress your immune system (immunosuppressants) may be combined with your initial medication. Medicines called azathioprine or mercaptopurine are most commonly used.

These medicines aren't suitable for everyone, so a blood test should be carried out to check if you can use them. If they are not suitable, an alternative immunosuppressant medication called methotrexate may be used.

Side effects of these immunosuppressants can include:

- nausea and vomiting
- increased vulnerability to infection
- feeling tired, breathless and weak, which is caused by anaemia (a decrease in the number of red blood cells)
- liver problems

During the course of medication you will have regular blood tests to check for serious side effects.

Azathioprine and mercaptopurine are not recommended during pregnancy or breastfeeding, but if you're already taking them your doctor may advise you to stay on them to prevent active inflammatory bowel disease – which may be a greater risk to you and the baby.

Methotrexate must not be taken for at least six months before trying for a baby (applies to both males and females) as this drug is know to cause birth defects. It must also be avoided while you are breastfeeding.

It's important to discuss the safety, risks and benefits of these medicines with your doctor, specialist nurse and your maternity team if you are or are planning to be pregnant or if you plan to breastfeed during the course of your treatment for Crohn's disease.

Severe Crohn's disease

For people in poor general health with severe symptoms of Crohn's disease, medicines called biological therapies may be used to reduce your symptoms if corticosteroids and immunosuppressants are unsuitable or ineffective.

Biological therapies are a type of powerful immunosuppressant medication created using naturally occurring biological substances, such as antibodies and enzymes.

The two medicines used to treat Crohn's disease in the UK are called infliximab and adalimumab. They work by targeting a protein called TNF-alpha (tumour necrosis factor-alpha), which is believed to be responsible for the inflammation associated with Crohn's disease.

Infliximab can be used for children over six years old and adults, but adalimumab should only be used for adults.

Infliximab is given as a drip into a vein in your arm (known as infusion) in hospital. Adalimumab is given as an injection and it may be possible for you, a family member or a friend to be taught how to give it so you don't need to visit hospital for every treatment.

Treatment will usually last at least 12 months, unless they stop being effective sooner than this. After this time, your condition will be assessed to determine if further treatment is necessary.

There is a risk of these medicines causing an allergic reaction, which can cause symptoms such as:

- itchy skin
- high temperature
- joint and muscle pain
- swelling of the hands or lips
- problems swallowing

You should seek immediate medical assistance if you experience these symptoms. Reactions can occur immediately after treatment, although they have been known to occur months later, even after treatment stops.

Surgery

Surgery may be recommended to reduce your symptoms if your healthcare team feel the benefits outweigh the risks.

In many cases, a type of surgery called a resection is used. This involves removing the inflamed area of the intestine and stitching the healthy sections together.

In some cases, your doctor may recommend a procedure called an ileostomy to temporarily divert digestive waste away from the inflamed colon (large intestine) to give it a chance to heal. During this operation, the end of the small intestine (the ileum) is disconnected from the colon and re-routed through a hole made in the abdomen, which is known as a stoma. An external bag is attached to the opening to collect waste products.

Once the colon has sufficiently recovered - usually after several months - a second operation will be needed to close the stoma and re-attach the small intestine to the colon.

Maintaining remission

Remission is a period when you don't have any symptoms, or your symptoms are mild. During these periods, you can choose whether or not to use medication to help maintain this.

If you decide not to have further treatment, you should be advised about attending regular follow-up appointments, and which symptoms to look out for. These include unintended weight loss, abdominal pain and diarrhoea.

If you choose treatment, this will usually involve immunosuppressants. Corticosteroids are not recommended for maintaining remission.

2.4.1 Complications of Crohn's disease

People with Crohn's disease are at risk of developing a number of complications.

The two most common problems associated with Crohn's disease are discussed in more detail below.

Intestinal stricture

The inflammation of the bowel (intestines) in Crohn's disease can cause scar tissue to form, leading to the affected areas becoming narrowed. This is known as stricture.

If this happens, there is a risk of digestive waste causing an obstruction, This means you will not be able to pass any stools, or you will only be able to pass watery stools.

Other symptoms of bowel obstruction include:

- abdominal pain and cramping
- being sick (vomiting)
- bloating
- an uncomfortable feeling of fullness in your abdomen

Left untreated, there is a risk that the bowel should split (rupture). This creates a hole that the contents of the bowel can leak from.

Intestinal stricture is usually treated with surgery to widen the affected section of intestine. In some cases, this may be achieved using a procedure called balloon dilation which is performed during colonoscopy (see diagnosing Crohn's disease for more information). During balloon dilation, a colonoscope is passed up your back passage (rectum) and a balloon inserted through the colonoscope. This is then inflated to open up the affected area.

If this doesn't work or is unsuitable, a surgical procedure known as a stricturoplasty may be needed to widen the affected area. During this operation, the surgeon widens the narrowed part of the intestine by opening it, reshaping it and sewing it back together.

Fistulas

If your digestive system becomes scarred due to excessive inflammation, ulcers can develop.

Over time the ulcers develop into tunnels, or passageways, that run from one part of your digestive system to another or, in some cases, to the bladder, vagina, anus or skin. These passageways are known as fistulas.

Small fistulas do not usually cause symptoms. However, larger fistulas can become infected and cause symptoms such as:

- a constant, throbbing pain
- a high temperature (fever) of 38°C (100°F) or above
- blood or pus in your faeces (stools)
- leakage of stools or mucus into your underwear

If a fistula develops on your skin (usually on, or near, the anus) it may release a foul-smelling discharge.

A type of medication called biological medication is usually used to treat fistulas, when these are not effective surgery is usually required. Read more about treating a fistula.

Other complications

People with Crohn's disease are also at an increased risk of other complications, such as:

- osteoporosis - weakening of the bones caused by the intestines not absorbing nutrients and by the use of steroid medication to treat Crohn's disease
- iron deficiency anaemia - a condition that can occur in people with Crohn's disease due to bleeding in the digestive tract; common symptoms include tiredness, shortness of breath and a pale complexion

- vitamin B12 or folate deficiency anaemia - a condition caused by a lack of vitamin B12 or folate being absorbed by the body; common symptoms include tiredness and lack of energy
- pyoderma gangrenosum - a rare skin reaction that causes painful skin ulcers

Children with Crohn's disease may also experience problems with their growth and development, due to a lack of nutrients being absorbed by the body.

3   HOW TO HANDLE A CROHN'S FLARE-UP

Crohn's disease is a form of inflammatory bowel disease (IBD) that affects the body's digestive system, causing inflammation and irritation in the bowel and large intestine (colon). This results in symptoms like abdominal pain, cramping, severe diarrhea, weight loss, bloody stools, and fever.

Crohn's disease goes through periods of remission and periods in which the symptoms and inflammation suddenly reactivate, known as flare-ups (or flares). Flare-ups aren't always predictable, but they can be managed and treated with medication, dietary adjustments, and surgery.

What Triggers a Crohn's Flare-Up?

Crohn's flare-ups occur when symptoms reappear. Some factors that may trigger a flare-up include:

- Missing or mismanaging medication (skipping a dose or taking the wrong dose of prescribed medication)
- Taking nonsteroidal anti-inflammatory drugs (NSAIDs), like aspirin and ibuprofen
- Stress (physical or emotional)
- Smoking
- Taking antibiotics, which can cause diarrhea and inflammation
- Eating specific foods do not cause flare-ups, but they can make them worse if they irritate the digestive system.

Symptoms

Monitoring your symptoms can help you recognize and manage your Crohn's disease flare-ups.

Flare-up symptoms will vary based on the severity of each Crohn's case and the exact part of the digestive tract it affects, but common signs of a Crohn's flare-up include:

- Frequent or urgent bowel movements
- Diarrhea
- Bloody stool
- Abdominal pain and cramping
- Nausea and vomiting
- Weight loss
- Fatigue
- Loss of appetite
- Joint pain

- Fever

Crohn's symptoms can worsen as the disease progresses. But having a Crohn's flare doesn't automatically mean that your Crohn's disease is getting worse. Your healthcare provider can help determine whether the flare is due to an infection, a change in your body's response to medications, stress, antibiotic use, or another cause.

3.1 TREATMENT OPTIONS

Crohn's disease is chronic, which means that it is a long-term condition requiring ongoing care. While there's currently no cure, it can be managed with ongoing treatment.

Treatment options for Crohn's flare-ups can include:

- Medications

- Diet modifications

- Lifestyle adjustments

- Surgery

The goal of treatment is to get the flare under control.

How Long Does a Crohn's Flare Last?

Flare-ups can last for a few days or as long as a few months, depending on the severity of the Crohn's case.

Medications

Although medications do not cure Crohn's, they can provide symptom relief during a flare-up.

Some prescription medication options include:

- Corticosteroids help quickly reduce whole-body inflammation during flares. They're usually recommended for short-term use, as long-term use can cause potentially serious side effects like high blood pressure, glaucoma (eye conditions that damage the optic nerve), and osteoporosis (brittle bones).

- Aminosalicylates can help control inflammation on an ongoing basis, particularly in more mild cases of Crohn's. This class of medications can cause side effects like diarrhea, vomiting, and heartburn.

- Biologics help target the immune system inflammatory response, typically prescribed for patients with moderate-to-severe Crohn's disease who haven't responded to other forms of treatment. Common side effects include headache, fatigue, diarrhea, upper respiratory tract infection, and rash.

- Immunomodulators are a certain type of biologic drug (made from the cells of a living organism) that help cut down on inflammation. They're typically prescribed for people who have not responded to aminosalicylates or corticosteroids. Side effects can include fatigue, nausea, vomiting, pancreatitis, kidney impairment, and an increased risk of infection.

Take Medication as Prescribed

It's important to take all prescription medications consistently as directed by your healthcare providers to help prevent flare-ups. Even if your symptoms are mild, missing a dose can lead to a flare.

Over-the-counter (OTC) drug treatment options for Crohn's disease may also be used to help treat mild pain and diarrhea. These include:

- Tylenol (acetaminophen) may be recommended for mild pain relief rather than NSAIDs like aspirin, Aleve (naproxen), and Advil or Motrin (ibuprofen), as NSAIDs can cause gastrointestinal bleeding and ulcers.

- Antidiarrheal medications like Imodium (loperamide) can help slow bowel contractions and relieve short bouts of diarrhea. They're used short term under the direction of your healthcare provider, as overuse can lead to potentially serious side effects in the colon.

Dietary Adjustments

While a specific diet can't cure Crohn's, and there's no specific Crohn's flare-up diet, you may be able to manage flares by making some temporary changes to the way you eat. Because normal digestive processes can be stressful on your system, certain dietary adjustments can give your digestive system time to heal.

Your healthcare provider may recommend a registered dietician or nutritionist to develop a plan that works for you. Some options include:

- Low-fiber diet: High-fiber foods like raw vegetables and whole grains require your intestines to do more work. Simple, bland, low-fiber food like plain white rice, bananas, applesauce, gluten-free bread, and clear soups or broths are easier for your body to digest.

- Low-residue diet: Some foods leave less residue in your colon, leading to fewer bowel movements, which can be especially helpful during a flare. A low-residue diet involves cutting out foods like seeds, whole grains, raw vegetables, beans, cured meats, popcorn, and crunchy peanut butter. While experts say this may be one of the best ways to calm a Crohn's flare-up, you usually don't have to stick to this diet permanently.

- Liquid diet and bowel rest: In more serious circumstances, your healthcare provider may recommend temporarily consuming high-calorie liquid foods and nutritional shakes. This approach is often necessary after bowel surgery. Soft foods will later be introduced before you're able to tolerate solid foods again.

Tracking Food

To avoid putting any unnecessary stress on your digestive tract, consider tracking which foods negatively affect you. This helps identify foods you may need to cut back on.

Surgery

Many Crohn's patients will have surgery at some point, particularly those with moderate-to-severe cases of Crohn's that involve severe bowel obstruction, excessive bleeding, an abscess (pus-filled pocket), or an intestinal rupture (a hole that develops in the wall of the intestine).

Types of Crohn's surgery include:

Strictureplasty is a surgical technique used to widen a narrowed intestinal passage (known as a stricture).

Bowel resection involves the removal of part of the small intestine that is affected. It's often used when a stricture is too large to be treated with strictureplasty.

Colectomy is the removal of the entire colon, or the affected part of the colon. This procedure is recommended for severe cases.

Proctectomy involves removing the rectum and the anus. This means that another way will be needed for stool to leave the body, either through reattachment of the small intestine to the anus, or through a hole in the lower abdomen (known as an ileostomy).

Prevention

While there's no definitive way to predict a Crohn's disease flare-up, experts recommend implementing a few lifestyle measures to encourage healthy bowel function, rather than triggering inflammation.

Dietary adjustments: There is no scientific evidence that a poor diet causes Crohn's disease or Crohn's flare-ups. But experts say it's still helpful to avoid certain trigger foods (including fatty, sugary, or spicy foods, along with caffeine and alcohol) that could irritate your digestive system.

Exercise: Although Crohn's symptoms may make it challenging to be physically active, research shows that making low- to moderate-impact exercise a part of your regular routine can help prevent future flare-ups.

Stress management: Stress doesn't directly cause Crohn's disease, but it can impact your symptoms. This is why it's important to find stress management strategies that work for you. Some Crohn's patients use mind-body therapies, like meditation, deep breathing, tai chi, yoga, and biofeedback, to help prevent and treat flare-ups.

Quitting smoking: Smokers with Crohn's disease have a much higher risk of getting flares and are more likely to require aggressive immunosuppressant therapy compared to nonsmokers. If you need help quitting, your healthcare provider can recommend the smoking cessation options that are available to you.

Patient-physician communication: Maintaining regular communication with your healthcare provider and healthcare team can help make management and prevention of Crohn's flare-ups easier in the long run. Contact your healthcare provider at the first sign of a flare-up, because they can help identify the trigger and tweak your treatment plan as needed.

4 WHAT TO EAT WHEN YOU HAVE CROHN'S DISEASE

There's no single diet that works for everyone who has Crohn's disease. You may be able to manage a "flare" of symptoms by making some temporary changes to your diet.

Some people with Crohn's and other chronic gastrointestinal diseases find sticking to a certain diet even when they are not having symptoms helps manage their condition. Diet can be used as the first line of therapy or in combination therapy with medications for best results.

Peanut butter and banana on rice cakes, healthy, dietary food. Black background.

When you have Crohn's symptoms, avoiding certain foods and beverages may help you feel better. How you eat may also help prevent certain complications from Crohn's.

Research has shown that diet may have an effect on the progression of Crohn's. But ultimately there are many factors that determine whether a person gets Crohn's (particularly genetics).

According to research, some people with Crohn's report fewer flares if they regularly eat a high-fiber diet. However, you may feel better sticking to a low-fiber diet when you have symptoms.

How It Works

Some types of food are harder for your body to digest than others. Generally, high-fiber foods like raw vegetables and whole grains require your intestines to do more work than simple, bland, low-fiber food like plain white rice.

When your intestines are weak and damaged, normal digestive processes can be stressful. Asking your body to do a little less work gives your gastrointestinal tract time to heal.

Putting less demand on your intestines can also ease your symptoms. Some foods leave less residue in your colon, meaning you'll have fewer bowel movements which can be especially helpful if you're having diarrhea.

Avoiding other hard-to-digest foods like those that are high in fat, spicy, or sugary-sweet can also help reduce symptoms. Choosing foods that can pass through your digestive tract easily eliminates the stress of "heavy" foods. Keeping food bland also helps prevent more inflammation.

Duration

A Crohn's diet may take two forms. You may have one list of foods to eat when you aren't feeling well and another for when you are not having symptoms.

You may also choose to eat a consistent diet whether or not you are having symptoms if you feel certain foods help you control flares.

You will need to work with your healthcare provider to find a healthy, balanced, diet that works for you in the long term. A registered dietician or nutritionist may also be able to help.

In certain circumstances, your healthcare provider may make strict or specific dietary recommendations that are meant for a shorter period of time.

National Institute of Diabetes and Digestive and Kidney Diseases. Eating, diet, and nutrition for Crohn's disease.

For example, if you have bowel surgery you may be put on a liquid-only diet for the first few days of recovery. Your practitioner may suggest a soft diet to help you transition back to your normal diet.

What to Eat

There are general dietary guidelines you can follow, but some trial and error work will be necessary for you to create a personalized Crohn's diet tailored to your needs and tastes.

As you experiment with your diet you may find some foods make your symptoms worse. You may choose to avoid these "trigger" foods all the time or just when you're having a flare.

You'll also want to take note of which foods make you feel better (or at least, don't make you feel worse). "Safe" foods can be part of your regular and healing diet.

Compliant Foods

- Bananas
- Applesauce
- White rice
- Low-fat yogurt (as tolerated)
- Plain pasta noodles made from refined white flour
- Gluten-free bread
- Sourdough bread
- Saltines, rice crackers
- Smooth nut butter (as tolerated)

- Clear soups and broth

- White potato

- Chicken breast without skin, lean cut of pork

- Tofu

- Soft cooked eggs

- Honeydew melon, cantaloupe

Non-Compliant Foods

- Raw fruit with skin or seeds

- Prunes, prune juice

- Raw vegetables

- Corn

- Cruciferous vegetables (broccoli, cauliflower)

- Milk, cheese

- Lunchmeat

- Tough cuts of meat

- Wild rice, rice pilaf

- Cereal or granola with nuts/fruit

- Bran

- Dried fruit

- Butter, coconut, cream

- Chocolate

- Whole nuts

- Pastries, cakes, cookies, candy

- Popcorn

- Sugar substitutes such as xylitol and sorbitol

- Greasy, fatty, spicy, or fried foods

- Coffee

- Alcohol

Fruits and Vegetables: Fresh produce is an important part of a balanced, healthy diet. While raw fruits and veggies may be too irritating for your digestive system, many can be peeled, cut, and cooked to be easier to digest.

For example, a raw apple with the peel may have more fiber than your body can handle. Peeled, chopped, and cooked on the stove, applesauce is a diet staple for stomach upsets.

Vegetables like potato and squash are easy to cook. You can bake them, boil them, or even microwave them. Low fiber fruits and veggies can also be juiced or puréed for smoothies.

Some high-fiber fruits and veggies may be best avoided, as they can increase intestinal gas, such as corn, broccoli, and prunes.

Grains: When you're having symptoms, choose bread, pasta, and other carbohydrates made from refined white flour instead of whole grains.4 White rice is another low-fiber option. Avoid brown rice, wild rice, or rice pilaf.

Use sourdough bread for toast or, if you don't eat gluten, look for white bread style gluten-free loaves. Hot cereals, such as Cream of Wheat, may work well. Simply prepared packets of oatmeal are approved if you tolerate them. Avoid cereal and granola that has dried fruit, nuts, or other additions.

Dairy: Even if you aren't lactose intolerant milk products can be hard to digest during a flare-up of gastrointestinal symptoms. The only dairy products you may wish to include are low-fat yogurts that don't have added sugars. Yogurt is a good source of probiotics, which may benefit digestive health.

Protein: Choose lean sources of protein, such as skinless chicken breast. Avoid frying food or cooking with oil, butter, or spices. Be careful not to overcook the meat, you don't want it to be tough.

Plant-based protein staples like beans and legumes can cause gas. Tofu or tempeh may work as a non-meat protein source. Whole nuts can be difficult to digest but you may tolerate small portions of smooth nut butter.

Desserts: Avoid rich, sugary, fatty treats like cakes, cookies, ice cream, pudding. Gelatin may be OK, but don't add any whipped topping. Be sure to look out for and avoid sugar substitutes like xylitol and sorbitol in "sugar-free" products, especially hard candy and gum. These ingredients sometimes cause digestive distress.

Beverages: You'll want to do your best to stay hydrated, but you may find carbonated beverages, caffeine, and alcohol worsen your symptoms. Stick to water, electrolyte-replacement drinks, or nutritional supplements recommended by your healthcare provider.

Recommended Timing

When you're having symptoms, you may find you feel better eating smaller amounts more frequently throughout the day as opposed to sitting down to three big meals.3 You may feel the best eating on this schedule even when you are not having symptoms.

If you tend to get uncomfortably full quickly, try having drinks and meals or snacks separately.

Modifications

You can make adjustments to the Crohn's diet to accommodate special dietary needs, food allergies, or other medical conditions.

If you're pregnant, you might experience flares, though many people experience fewer Crohn's symptoms during pregnancy.5 You might need to modify the Crohn's diet to ensure you are able to manage your Crohn's symptoms—as well as any pregnancy symptoms and still staying properly nourished.

Children can also have Crohn's. Like adults, they may need to be on a certain diet to manage the condition. The dietary needs of children and young adults are very important because growth and development are tied to nutritional status. Kids and teens with Crohn's may need nutritional supplementation to prevent malnourishment, especially if they resist eating due to pain.

Research indicates special diets used to treat digestive disorders, such as the Specific

Carbohydrate Diet, may be helpful for children with Crohn's.

Considerations

You can work with your healthcare provider, nutritionist, and other members of your healthcare team to figure out how making changes to your diet to manage Crohn's relates to other aspects of your life.

The responsibilities you have at home, work, or school, as well as your social life, can both affect your ability to follow a specific diet and require you to make changes to your lifestyle. Understanding how other factors influence your Crohn's diet plan will be an essential part of finding a routine that works for you.

General Nutrition

It can be difficult to get adequate nutrition if you need to limit your diet or avoid certain food groups. If you're having a hard time eating enough on a Crohn's diet, your healthcare provider may suggest you try liquid nutritional supplements.

If your Crohn's is severe and causes you to become malnourished, your healthcare provider may want you to have a feeding tube to help restore nutrition.

Dietary Restrictions

If you have other dietary considerations, such as needing to avoid gluten due to celiac disease, or preferring a plant-based diet, talk to your healthcare provider or nutritionist about how you can make these needs and preferences work for a Crohn's diet.

For example, many gluten-free brands of bread and pasta come in the style of white bread rather than multigrain or wheat. If you're looking for gluten-free pasta noodles, avoid alternatives made with beans, legumes, and corn.

If you're vegan or vegetarian, you may already be avoiding some foods that are not compliant with a Crohn's diet. However, many staples of plant-based diets, including whole grains, beans, and raw produce, are not approved. If your diet becomes too restricted, you may have a hard time getting the nutrition you need.

You'll need to work with your healthcare team to adjust your diet according to these preferences while still managing your Crohn's symptoms. You may need to take vitamins or other supplements to prevent deficiencies.

Support and Community

If you have Crohn's disease you may already be part of an in-person or online support community for patients. If you have questions or concerns about changing your diet to manage the condition, you should talk to your healthcare provider. However, it can often be helpful to talk to other people who have "been there" and will understand what you're going through on an emotional level.

When you are feeling ill or recovering from a procedure, try your best to let family and friends help you. You can prepare a lot of Crohn's diet-friendly meals ahead of time and freeze them, but it will be a big help if you have someone who can heat food up for you or run to the store for cold drinks, crackers, or to pick up prescriptions.

Cost

Many of the foods suitable for a Crohn's diet (such as white rice) are affordable, especially if you buy them in bulk.

Kitchen implements like blenders or handheld food processors can make pureeing foods for a Crohn's diet much easier. You can certainly find more expensive tools, but a basic blender will do the job for about $20. You can also find other affordable options online.

While you can buy many brands of liquid supplemental nutrition (such as Ensure) at the grocery store or pharmacy, they can be expensive. If your healthcare provider wants you to include them in your diet, ask if they can be prescribed. If you have insurance, these products (or similar products) may be covered by your plan.

Side Effects

Some temporary digestive upset is common whenever you make changes to your diet. Eating more or less of certain foods, especially those with fiber, can directly affect your bowel function (both in terms of the consistency or quality of your bowel movements as well as how frequent they are).

While these symptoms will likely get better as your body adjusts to your new diet, let your healthcare provider know if they persist or get worse. Constipation from a low-fiber diet may benefit from fiber supplements or something as simple as drinking more water throughout the day. Diarrhea that doesn't get better after a few days may be a sign of an underlying condition and also puts you at risk for becoming dehydrated.

Energy and General Health

If you're eating less solid food or focusing on primarily bland foods to manage a flare of Crohn's symptoms, you may find you don't have as much energy as you typically do.

Make it your goal to get as much nutrition as you can every day, which includes eating enough calories to fuel your body. Adequate nutrition from a varied, balanced, diet isn't just important for managing Crohn's. it's also important to maintaining your overall health.

If you have Crohn's you're at risk for complications from the disease, including infections. You may also be more likely to have other health conditions, some of which may be linked to your immune system.

Proper nourishment is one way you can help your body heal from a Crohn's flare as well as any other ailments you're trying to manage.

5   Meal Plan for Crohn's Disease

Your meal plan (when you are in remission) should include foods that help you feel your best. When managing Crohn's disease, you may need to make texture modifications to your meal to help with digestion. For example, peeling an apple before eating it or cooking carrots instead of eating them raw.

Below is an example of a 7-day meal plan for Crohn's disease that you can modify to satisfy your preferences. The meals listed below should be adjusted to meet your serving size requirements. If you need help figuring out how much food is enough for you, consider booking a virtual appointment with a Nourish dietitian.

Day 1

- Breakfast - Oatmeal cooked in skim milk (use lactose-free or a plant-based alternative if better tolerated), topped with fresh raspberries, roasted almonds, and lemon zest. You can add a drizzle of honey if desired.

- Lunch - Chicken noodle soup with carrots, parsnip, and fresh parsley. Add a side of strawberries to enjoy after your meal.

- Dinner - Sheet pan meal with baked extra firm tofu, butternut squash, and green beans. Drizzle with garlic-infused oil and serve over rice.

- Snacks - hard-boiled egg with baked crackers and sliced red pepper; peach slices and ground cinnamon served over lactose-free cottage cheese.

Day 2

- Breakfast - Toasted sourdough bread with light cream cheese, smoked salmon, and freshly cut red onion. Drizzle with fresh lemon juice before eating.

- Lunch - Lettuce wraps with ground turkey, avocado slices, fresh tomato, cheddar cheese, and a tangy tahini dressing. Enjoy pineapple slices on the side for extra vitamins and carbohydrates (an essential energy source.)

- Dinner - BBQ chicken skewers served with baked potatoes. Add a fresh salad with romaine lettuce, cucumber, tomato, red onion, olives, and a sprinkle of feta cheese. Dress with a simple olive oil and lemon juice vinaigrette.

- Snacks - Toasted whole wheat pita triangles with hummus; baked apple with cinnamon and lactose-free plain Greek yogurt.

Day 3

- Breakfast - Scrambled eggs with spinach, diced tomato, feta cheese, and fresh basil. Serve with a side of whole-grain toast.

- Lunch - Olive oil-based tuna salad with fresh basil, sun dried tomatoes, and sweet onion. Serve on a whole-grain bun.

- Dinner - Ground turkey meatballs made with mint, served over pasta with grilled zucchini and your favorite red sauce.

- Snacks - Banana with nut butter; avocado dip with baked crackers.

Day 4

- Breakfast - Green smoothie with kale, extra soft tofu, banana, blueberries, ground flax seeds, and a spoonful of your favorite nut butter.

- Lunch - Hearty baby arugula salad with canned salmon, cooked sweet potato, caramelized onions, and cucumber. Dress with olive oil and balsamic vinaigrette - add fresh chopped sage to increase the flavor.

- Dinner - Grilled salmon served with fresh mango salsa - made with diced white onions, lime juice, and cilantro. Serve over boiled quinoa with a side of steamed green beans and carrots.

- Snacks - Roasted chickpeas with fresh fruit on the side; homemade kale chips dressed with nutritional yeast.

Day 5

- Breakfast - Overnight oatmeal with skim milk (use lactose-free or a plant-based alternative if better tolerated), peeled diced apples, cinnamon, and a dollop of walnut butter.

- Lunch - Mid-day egg frittata made with shredded zucchini, bell peppers, oregano, and goat cheese. Serve with a side of toast.

- Dinner - Individual pizzas made with whole wheat pita bread, chicken sausage slices, pesto, kale, and shallots. Serve with a side salad made with your favorite vegetables.

- Snacks - Charcuterie-style snack with fresh fruits and cheese slices - add your favorite baked crackers; cucumber slices with roasted red pepper dip.

- Day 6

- Breakfast - Whole grain wrap with avocado, arugula, fresh tomato, chopped hard-boiled egg, cheese, and Dijon mustard.

- Lunch - A grainy bowl with wheatberry, grilled chicken, fresh lettuce, tomato, sliced avocado, and a dollop of chunky salsa.

- Dinner - Shrimp stir fry with cooked bell peppers, onion, baby bok choy leaves, and a homemade sauce with sesame oil, ginger, orange juice, and grated garlic. Serve over rice.

- Snacks - Plain lactose-free yogurt dressed with fresh fruit; baked crackers with cheese.

Day 7

- Breakfast - Whole grain toast with smooth peanut butter and fresh banana slices, sprinkled with dark chocolate chips and ground cinnamon.

- Lunch - Barley soup with frozen carrots, peas, and turkey. Serve with a side of your favorite fresh fruit.

- Dinner - Breakfast for dinner! Enjoy pan-fried eggs over toast, add fresh cantaloupe on the side, and a baby arugula salad with blueberries, cucumber, and tomato.

- Snacks - Cherry tomatoes with beet hummus; no-bake oatmeal power balls made with quick oats, peanut butter, dried cranberries, and maple syrup.

Tips for Meal Preparation

A few common barriers to consistent meal preparation include a lack of access to certain foods, a decreased availability of vegetables (which can be affected by your income), a lack of confidence in cooking skills, and not having a supportive home environment that promotes healthy eating. Fortunately, there are small solutions that can help make meal preparation easier.

Frozen vegetables and fruits can be more affordable, and their nutritional value is on par with fresh varieties.

Buy precut vegetables to save you valuable time in the kitchen. They might be slightly more expensive, but if it helps you eat vegetables regularly, they can be worth the extra dollars.

Batch cook your dishes whenever possible. You can freeze the leftovers and simply reheat them in the future for a quick meal.

Visit local farmer's markets to gain access to various foods that are in season. You may have more options available to you compared to big box grocery stores.

Schedule a day and time in your week for meal planning and preparation. Creating this routine can help you build the habit, which should feel easier over time.

Talk to your family members about your health goals and ask for support. Chances are everyone in the house will benefit from these nutrition-conscious changes!

6.1   MACADAMIA–CHOCOLATE CHIP COOKIES

Ingredients

8 tablespoons unsalted butter, cut into cubes, at room temperature ¼ cup packed light brown sugar

¼ cup superfine sugar 1 large egg

1 teaspoon vanilla extract

2/3 cup superfine white rice flour ½ cup cornstarch

¼ cup soy flour

½ teaspoon baking soda

½ cup (95 g) chocolate chips

½ cup (70 g) roasted unsalted macadamia nuts, roughly chopped

Instructions

Preheat the oven to 325 degrees Fahrenheit (170 degrees Celsius). Preheat oven to 350°F. Line two baking pans with parchment paper. Use a hand-held electric mixer to thoroughly combine the butter, brown sugar, and superfine sugar in a medium mixing bowl until they are thick and pale. The egg and vanilla essence should be beaten together in a separate basin. Sift the rice flour, cornstarch, soy flour, and baking soda three times in a mixing dish (or whisk in the bowl until well combined). Add the macadamia nuts and chocolate chips to the butter mixture and whisk until well combined. Spread out adequate room on the sheets before dropping spoonfuls of dough there. Bake for 10 - 15 minutes, or up to golden brown, in a 350°F oven. Cool on the sheets for five minutes before moving to a wire rack to finish cooling.

6.2   ALMOND COOKIES

Ingredients

3/4 cup almond flour

1 tablespoon plus 1 teaspoon cornstarch ½ teaspoon

gluten-free baking powder 1 large egg white

½ cup superfine sugar

1 teaspoon finely grated lemon zest 3 drops almond

extract

1 tablespoon unsalted butter, melted

Instructions

Set the oven heat to 275 degrees Fahrenheit (140 degrees Celsius). Set the oven to 350°F. Using parchment paper, line two baking pans. Almond flour, cornstarch, and baking powder should all be combined in a small mixing basin. With a hand-held electric mixer, whip the egg whites in a clean medium basin until soft peaks form. Incorporate the sugar gradually. Beat for a another five minutes, or until stiff peaks develop. Melted butter, lemon zest, almond essence, and the combination of almond flour should be added gradually with a large metal spoon. Using two teaspoons of dough, form a ball. With the remaining dough, form about 40 balls, and arrange them on the baking sheets with some space between them for spreading. Flatten a little. 25 minutes of baking is required to get a light golden hue. Cool on the sheets for five minutes before moving to a wire rack to finish cooling.

6.3   PEANUT BUTTER AND SESAME COOKIES

Ingredients

2 tablespoons unsalted butter, at room temperature

1 cup creamy peanut butter

1/4 cup packed light brown sugar

2 heaping tablespoons superfine sugar 2 large eggs, lightly beaten

1 teaspoon vanilla extract 1/4 cup sesame seeds

2/3 cup superfine white rice flour 3/4 cup cornstarch

1/2 cup soy flour

1/2 teaspoon baking soda

1 teaspoon xanthan gum or guar gum

Instructions

Turn the oven's temperature up to 350 degrees (170 degrees Celsius). Set the oven to 350°F. Using parchment paper, line two baking pans. Use a hand-held electric mixer to thoroughly blend the butter, peanut butter, brown sugar, and superfine sugar in a medium mixing bowl. Well combine the sesame seeds, vanilla, and eggs. Sift the rice flour, cornstarch, soy flour, baking soda, and xanthan gum three times in a large mixing basin (or whisk in the bowl until well combined). With a large metal spoon, add to the peanut butter mixture and stir until well combined. Create dough balls the size of walnuts, and then arrange them on the baking sheets with sufficient room between them for spreading. gently flatten until it is about 14 inches thick (5 mm). Bake for 10 to 12 minutes, or until golden brown, in a 350°F oven. Cool on the sheets for five minutes before moving to a wire rack to finish cooling.

6.4   HAZELNUT OR ALMOND CRESCENTS

Ingredients

⅓ cup superfine white rice flour, plus more for the work surface ¼ cup cornstarch

¼ cup superfine sugar

1¼ cups hazelnut or almond flour

7 tablespoons unsalted butter, cut into cubes, at room temperature 1 large egg yolk, at room temperature, lightly beaten

1 teaspoon vanilla extract

½ cup confectioners' sugar, plus more for dusting

Instructions

Sift together the rice flour and cornstarch in a medium mixing basin (or whisk in the bowl until well combined). In a mixing dish, combine the hazelnut flour and ultrafine sugar. When the mixture resembles bread crumbs, work the butter into it with your hands. Fold the egg yolk and vanilla essence in with a large metal spoon. Rice flour may be used to gently dust your work surface. The dough should be rolled into a smooth ball, which you should then set on a board that has been floured. The dough needs to be split into two equal pieces before being plastic-wrapped.Refrigerate for 15 minutes. While the dough chills, preheat the oven to 325°F (160°C). Set the oven to 350°F. Using parchment paper, line two baking pans. Take the dough out of the packaging, then roll each piece into a 34-inch log (2 cm). With your hands, make slices that are 34 to 1 inch (2 to 3 cm) wide and shape them into round crescents. Place on baking sheets with sufficient space between them to for spreading. Until golden brown, bake for 15 to 20 minutes. Allow the sheets to cool for five minutes.

Sift the confectioners' sugar into a little plate (or whisk well in the bowl). After thoroughly coating the warm cookies in sugar, lay them aside to cool completely on a wire rack. Dust with extra confectioners' sugar right before serving.

6.5 AMARETTI

Ingredients

1 cup almond flour (preferably finely ground)

3/4 cup confectioners' sugar

1 tablespoon plus 1 teaspoon cornstarch 2 large egg whites

1/3 cup superfine sugar

1 teaspoon almond extract

Instructions

Set the oven heat to 325 degrees Fahrenheit (170 degrees Celsius). Set the oven to 350°F. I am using parchment paper and lining two baking pans.

Combine the almond flour, confectioners' sugar, and cornstarch in a medium mixing basin. I use a handheld electric mixer to whisk the egg whites in a clean, medium mixing bowl until soft peaks form. Superfine sugar should be added one tablespoon at a time while beating the mixture to make glossy, firm peaks. The almond extract should be added and well mixed. The almond flour mixture should be carefully folded using a large metal spoon until barely incorporated. Give them room to spread when you drop rounded teaspoons of batter onto the baking sheets. Smooth the tops of each biscuit with the back of a metal spoon. Until golden brown, bake for 18 to 25 minutes. After the oven is turned off and the door is left ajar, let the cookies cool and dry inside.

6.6 BANANA FRIANDS (MINI ALMOND CAKES)

Ingredients

9 tablespoons unsalted butter, cut into cubes

1¼ cups confectioners' sugar, plus more for dusting

¼ cup cornstarch

¼ cup superfine white rice flour 1¼ cups almond flour

5 large egg whites, lightly beaten

1 tablespoon plus 1 teaspoon fresh lemon juice 1 teaspoon vanilla extract

1 small ripe banana, peeled and roughly chopped

Instructions

Turn the oven's temperature to 350 degrees (180 degrees Celsius). Lightly oil a 12-cup muffin pan, fry pan, or small loaf pan with cooking spray. Melt the butter in a small skillet over low heat, then cook for

3 to 4 minutes, or until brown specks appear. Take it out of the equation. Sift the rice flour, cornstarch, and confectioners' sugar three times in a large mixing basin (or whisk in the bowl until well combined). Using a large metal spoon, stir in the almond flour before incorporating the egg whites, lemon juice, vanilla, and melted butter. Add the pieces of banana and mix thoroughly. Fill each cup with the batter until they are two-thirds full. Bake for 12 - 15 minutes until firm and lightly golden (a toothpick inserted into the center should come out clean). Cool the cake in the pan for five minutes before transferring it to a wire rack to finish cooling. Just before serving, dust with confectioners' sugar.

6.7   BERRY FRIANDS (MINI ALMOND CAKES)

Ingredients

Nonstick cooking spray

9 tablespoons unsalted butter, cut into cubes

1½ cups confectioners' sugar, plus more for dusting

¼ cup cornstarch

¼ cup superfine white rice flour 1¼ cups almond flour

5 large egg whites, lightly beaten

1 tablespoon plus 1 teaspoon fresh lemon juice 2 teaspoons vanilla extract

1 cup blueberries or raspberries

Instructions

Turn the oven's temperature up to 350 degrees (180 degrees Celsius). Lightly oil a 12-cup muffin pan, friand pan, or small loaf pan with cooking spray. Melt the butter in a small skillet over low heat, then cook for a further 3 to 4 minutes, or until brown flecks appear. Take it out of the equation. Sift the rice flour, cornstarch, and confectioners' sugar three times in a large mixing basin (or whisk in the bowl until well combined). Using a large metal spoon, stir in the almond flour before incorporating the egg whites, lemon juice, vanilla, and melted butter. Fill each cup with the batter until they are two-thirds full. Gently push 4 berries into the center of each friand (without pressing all the way into the batter). Bake for 12 - 15 minutes, or until firm and light golden (a toothpick inserted into the center should come out clean). Cool in the pan for five minutes before transferring to a wire rack to finish cooling. Dust with confectioners' sugar just before serving.

6.8 BANANA FRITTERS WITH FRESH PINEAPPLE

Ingredients

1 cup dried gluten-free, soy-free bread crumbs* 1/3 cup packed light brown sugar

1 tablespoon ground cinnamon 2 large eggs

1/2 teaspoon confectioners' sugar

4 small bananas, peeled and halved lengthwise 2 tablespoons unsalted butter

Gluten-free, lactose-free vanilla ice cream, for serving ½ small pineapple, peeled, cored, and finely chopped Pulp of 2 passion fruits (optional)

Instructions

Set the oven to 300 degrees Fahrenheit. In a large dish, mix the cinnamon, brown sugar, and bread crumbs. In a small bowl, lightly whisk the eggs with the confectioners' sugar. After dipping the banana halves in the egg mixture, cover them well with the bread crumbs. Over medium-low temperature, melt 1 tablespoon of the butter in a large nonstick frying pan. Cook the first half of the banana slices for 3 to 4 minutes on each side, or until they are golden brown. Place on a baking pan, then reheat in the oven. Cook the remaining banana halves in the same manner, using the remaining 1 tablespoon butter. On four plates, distribute two banana halves each. Add ice cream, pineapple, and passion fruit pulp as garnishes (if desired). Serve right away.

6.9 SHORTBREAD FINGERS

Ingredients

1 cup confectioners' sugar

1 tablespoon plus 2 teaspoons vanilla sugar, plus more for sprinkling 2 cups cornstarch, plus more for kneading

1 cup soy flour

1/2 cup superfine white rice flour

2 teaspoons xanthan gum or guar gum

17 tablespoons unsalted butter, cut into cubes, at room temperature

Instructions

Set the oven heat to 275 degrees Fahrenheit (130 degrees Celsius). Set the oven to 350°F. Using parchment paper, line two baking pans. Confectioners' sugar, vanilla sugar, cornstarch, soy flour, rice flour, and xanthan gum should all be properly combined in a food processor or blender. Add the butter and process for an additional 3 to 5 minutes to create a dough. Dust your work surface lightly with cornstarch. The dough should come together once you turn it out onto the work area and gently knead it. The dough should be rolled out between two sheets of parchment paper to a thickness of 12 inches (1.25 cm). Place in two by 34-inch (5 x 2 cm) rectangles on baking sheets, leaving some space between each for spreading. On top, more vanilla sugar can be added. Bake for 20 - 25 minutes, or until golden brown, in a 200°F oven. Once the cookies are golden brown, lower the oven temperature to 200°F (100°C) and bake for an additional 10 minutes. Cool on the sheets for 10 to

12 minutes before moving to a wire rack to finish cooling.

6.10 CARAMEL NUT BARS

Ingredients

Nonstick cooking spray

1/2 cup superfine white rice flour 1/4 cup potato flour

1/3 cup cornstarch

1/4 cup superfine sugar 1/4 teaspoon baking soda

1/4 teaspoon gluten-free baking powder 1 teaspoon xanthan gum or guar gum

4 tablespoons unsalted butter, cut into cubes, at room temperature 1 large egg, beaten

1 teaspoon vanilla extract

Nut Topping

1 cup packed light brown sugar

10 tablespoons (1 stick plus 2 tablespoons/150 g) unsalted butter, cut into cubes, at room temperature

⅓ cup light cream

3 tablespoons plus 1 teaspoon cornstarch

½ cup roasted unsalted pecans, roughly chopped

⅔ cup roasted unsalted Brazil nuts (skin on), roughly chopped ½ cup roasted unsalted macadamia nuts, halved

Instructions

Set the oven's temperature to 350°F (180°C). Use cooking spray to grease and line an 11 x 7-inch (28 x 18-cm) baking sheet with parchment paper, allowing an overhang on the two long sides to aid in lifting the bars afterwards. In a bowl, mix the cornstarch, rice flour, potato flour, superfine sugar, baking soda, baking powder, and xanthan gum three times (or whisk in the bowl until well combined). Using your fingertips, work the butter in. With a big metal spoon, blend the egg and vanilla after being added. Use your hands to gather the mixture into a ball as it starts to solidify more. Rolling out the dough between two sheets of parchment paper to a thickness of 1/4 inch (5 mm). Fit it gently into the pan's bottom and give it a fork prick all over. 10 minutes in the refrigerator. Bake the crust for 10 - 12 minutes, or until it is firm and just brown. But keep the oven running, and set aside to cool. To preparing the topping, melt the butter in a large saucepan over medium heat while stirring the brown sugar mixture until it boils. Once the mixture is smooth, turning off the heat and whisk in the cream and cornstarch. Add the macadamia, brazil, and pecan nuts. Reset the stovetop to medium heat and continue to stir the mixture until it boils. Once the mixture is thick and sticky, turn the heat down to low and simmer gently for an additional 2 to 3 minutes. After uniformly dotting the crust with the nut topping, bake the pie for 15 minutes, or until the topping is boiling. After transferring to a board, removing the parchment paper, and cutting into little (or giant!) pieces for serving, allow it to cool fully in the pan.

6.11 CHOCOLATE-MINT BARS

Ingredients

Nonstick cooking spray

8 tablespoons unsalted butter, cut into cubes, at room temperature

⅓ cup superfine sugar

½ cup superfine white rice flour

¼ cup soy flour ½ cup cornstarch

1 teaspoon xanthan gum or guar gum

2 heaping tablespoons unsweetened cocoa powder

Peppermint Filling

1 cup confectioners' sugar

One 8-ounce package reduced-fat cream cheese, at room temperature 3 to 4 teaspoons peppermint extract

½ cup plus 2 tablespoons vegetable shortening, melted

Chocolate Topping

4 ounces good-quality dark chocolate, broken into pieces 1 tablespoon plus 1 teaspoon light cream

3 scant tablespoons vegetable shortening

Instructions

Set the oven's temperature to 325°F (170°C). Apply nonstick cooking spray to an 11 x 7-inch (29 19 cm) baking sheet and line with parchment paper. Using an electric mixer, combining the butter and sugar in a medium bowl and beat until thick and pale. Sift the cocoa, cornstarch, xanthan gum, soy flour, rice flour, and three times into a separate bowl (or whisk in a bowl until well combined). With a sizable metal spoon, blend the addition with the butter and sugar that have been creamed. Form a loose ball and give it a quick knead in the bowl. Into the prepared pan, press the dough. Bake for 10 - 15 minutes, or up to golden. Place aside and allow to fully cool. Confectioners' sugar, cream cheese, and peppermint essence are combined to form the peppermint filling. This mixture is then well mixed with a handheld electric mixer. Shortening should be added, then beaten for one to two minutes until smooth. Refrigerate until firm after evenly distributing the mixture over the cookie shell. Dark chocolate, cream, and shortening should be put in a small saucepan and heated slowly while being stirred constantly to form the chocolate topping. Spread the chocolate coating over the peppermint filling after taking the pan out of the fridge. Slice into squares once chilled and ready to serve.

6.12 MACADAMIA NUT BROWNIES

Ingredients

Nonstick cooking spray

10 tablespoons unsalted butter, cut into cubes

10½ ounces good-quality dark chocolate, broken into pieces 1¼ cups packed light brown sugar

⅔ cup superfine white rice flour

¼ cup cornstarch

1 teaspoon xanthan gum or guar gum 3 large eggs

2 teaspoons vanilla extract ½ cup dark chocolate chips ½ cup light cream

¾ cup roughly chopped macadamia nuts (optional)

Instructions

Set the oven temperature to 325 degrees Fahrenheit (160 degrees Celsius). An 11 x 7-inch (29 x 19-cm) baking pan with cooking spray should be lined with parchment paper. Melt the butter and chocolate together over low heat in a medium saucepan, stirring regularly until smooth. The brown sugar should be added and thoroughly mixed up. Allow cooling in a large mixing bowl to room temperature. Rice flour, cornstarch, and xanthan gum should be sifted three times into a separate basin (or whisked in a bowl until well combined). One at a time, whisk each egg into the chocolate mixture. Combine the sifted flour, vanilla, chocolate chips, cream, and macadamia nuts in a mixing bowl (if using). Scoop into the baking pan, and level the top after thoroughly mixing. Bake for another 20 to 25 minutes, or until just firm, while covered with foil after 20 minutes of baking. Once the pan has reached room temperature, remove it from the oven. For at least two to three hours, or even overnight, until firm. Remove the parchment paper, turn it out onto a cutting board, and cut into squares for serving.

6.13 CHOCOLATE TRUFFLES

Ingredients

7 ounces gluten-free vanilla cookies, finely crushed (about 2 cups) 1/3 cup unsweetened cocoa powder

1/3 cup sweetened condensed milk

2 tablespoons rum or brandy (optional) 1 1/2 cups gluten-free chocolate sprinkles

Instructions

The crushed cookies and cocoa should be combined in a medium mixing bowl. With your hands, combine the condensed milk and rum (if using) until a firm dough forms.

Pour the chocolate sprinkles into a small dish. Make balls out of teaspoons of the truffle mixture using your hands. Add the chocolate sprinkles to coat. Refrigerate the mixture until it becomes firm.

GINGERBREAD MEN

Ingredients

1 large egg

1/3 cup superfine sugar 1/2 cup brown rice syrup

5 tablespoons unsalted butter, melted 1 cup superfine white rice flour

1/2 cup potato flour 1 cup soy flour

1 teaspoon xanthan gum or guar gum 1 teaspoon gluten-free baking powder

1 to 11/2 heaping tablespoons ground ginger Cornstarch, for rolling out dough

Gluten-free icing (optional)

Instructions

Turn the oven's temperature up to 300 degrees (150 degrees Celsius). Set the oven to 350°F. Use parchment paper to line three baking pans (or work in batches). Use a wooden spoon to whisk the egg and sugar in a large mixing bowl. In a mixing dish, combine the melted butter and brown rice syrup. Sift the rice flour, potato flour, soy flour, xanthan gum, baking powder, and ginger three times in a separate bowl (or whisk in a bowl until well combined). To fully integrate into the syrup mixture, stir vigorously. Allow the mixture to chill for 15 minutes so that it may start to thicken. Dust your work surface lightly with cornstarch. On a floured board, roll out the dough to a thickness of 34 to 1 inch (2 to 3 mm). Use a cookie cutter to cut out any desired shapes, such as stars, pine trees, or anything else. Place on baking sheets with sufficient space between them to for spreading. Bake for 8 to 10 minutes in the oven at 350 degrees. Cool on the sheets for 10 to 15 minutes before moving to a wire rack to finish cooling.

Once the cake has cooled, you can add a gluten-free icing garnish if you choose.

6.14 CHOCOLATE SAUCE

Ingredients

Crème Filling:

1 cup superfine white rice flour

1 teaspoon xanthan gum or guar gum 1 heaping tablespoon sugar

3 large eggs

Crème Custard

2 cups low-fat milk, lactose-free milk, or suitable plant-based milk 6 large egg yolks

½ cup superfine sugar ⅓ cup cornstarch

2 teaspoons vanilla extract

Chocolate Custard

1/3 cup cornstarch

2 1/2 cups low-fat milk, lactose-free milk, or suitable plant-based milk 3 1/2 teaspoons sugar

4 ounces good-quality dark chocolate, broken into small pieces

2 tablespoons plus 2 teaspoons coffee liqueur or brewed strong espresso mixed with a bit ofunsweetened cocoa powder

1/2 teaspoon vanilla extract

Chocolate Sauce

4 ounces good-quality dark chocolate, broken into pieces 1/3 cup light cream

Instructions

Turn the oven's temperature to 400 degrees (200 degrees Celsius). Set the range to 350°F. I am using parchment paper and lining two baking pans. In a medium saucepan, bring the butter and 34 cups (185 ml) of water to a boil. Rice flour and xanthan gum should be mixed thoroughly in a bowl before being added to the pan and swiftly stirred. The batter will form a smooth ball and draw away from the pan's sides. The dough should be put in a medium mixing bowl. Using a handheld electric mixer, incorporate the sugar. Beat in the eggs one at a time. Place the dough on the sheets in rounded tablespoons, spacing them 112 inches (4 cm) apart. Bake the pastries for 7 minutes, or until they bubble up, in a 350°F oven. Bake for ten minutes, or until crisp and lightly browned, at 350 degrees Fahrenheit (180 degrees Celsius). One sheet should be removed from the oven after lowering the temperature to 275 degrees Fahrenheit (140 degrees Celsius). Quickly and carefully score a small hole in the side of each pastry. Repeat the technique with the second sheet after replacing the first one in the oven. The pies should be dried out after five minutes in the oven.

After taking it out of the oven, let it cool to room temperature. Carefully cut the pastries open. Without crushing them, remove the soft cores from the pastry cases. While the pastries are cooling, pour the milk into a small, heavy-bottomed pot and heat over medium until it just begins to boil. Utilizing a handheld electric mixer, beat the egg yolks and ultrafine sugar in a sizable mixing bowl until thick and creamy. Mix thoroughly after adding the cornstarch. The hot milk and cream should be well whipped together. When you add the mixture to the pan, stir it slowly over low heat until the custard has thickened. Add the vanilla essence after turning off the heat in the pan. The mixture should be poured into a bowl, covered, and chilled for one to two hours, or until it is very cold. To make the chocolate custard, combine the cornstarch with 12 cups (125 ml) of milk and whisk until completely smooth. The remaining 2 cups (500 mL) of milk and sugar should be heated in a small saucepan until just boiling. The custard will thicken as you gradually add the cornstarch mixture while stirring continuously. The liquid should be thick when it is ready to be removed from the heat. Whisk in the chocolate, coffee liqueur, and vanilla until smooth, and the chocolate has melted. The mixture should be poured into a bowl, covered, and chilled for one to two hours, or until it is very cold. In a heatproof dish or on top of a double boiler, mix the chocolate and cream to produce the chocolate sauce. Whisk the mixture while it is placed over a pot of boiling water or the base of a double boiler once the chocolate has melted and the cream is thoroughly integrated. Pour the contents half of which should be crème custard, and the other half should be chocolate custard into each pastry after carefully opening it. Add a dollop of warm chocolate sauce on top before serving.

6.15 COCONUT RICE PUDDING

Ingredients

3/4 cup superfine sugar

3 cups milk, lactose-free milk, or suitable plant-based milk (more if needed) One 13.5-ounce can light coconut milk

2 teaspoons vanilla extract 11/2 cups Arborio rice

Heaping 1/4 cup shredded sweetened or unsweetened coconut Maple syrup, for serving (optional)

Instructions

Bring the sugar, milk, coconut milk, and vanilla to a boil in a medium saucepan over medium-high heat, stirring often. Incorporate the rice. Abate the temperature to low and simmer for about 50 minutes, or until the liquid has been absorbed and the rice is mushy. Add additional milk if necessary.Meanwhile, preheat the oven to 325°Fahrenheit (170°C) and line a baking sheet with foil. On a baking sheet sprinkled with coconut, bake for 10-12 minutes, or until golden brown. Top the rice pudding with toasted coconut and a drizzle of maple syrup, if desired, and serve warm or at room temperature.

6.16 CHOCOLATE SOUFFLÉS

Ingredients

Nonstick cooking spray 1¼ cups superfine sugar

8 ounces good-quality dark chocolate, broken into pieces ½ cup light cream

6 large eggs, separated ⅔ cup cornstarch

¼ cup packed light brown sugar

½ cup low-fat milk, lactose-free milk, or suitable plant-based milk Confectioners' sugar, sifted (optional)

Instructions

Turn the oven's temperature to 350 degrees (180 degrees Celsius). Grease six 8-ounce (250 ml) soufflé dishes with cooking spray. Each dish should get one tablespoon of superfine sugar, which should be liberally covered and any surplus removed. In a heat-resistant bowl or the top of a double boiler, mix the chocolate and cream. Whisk the mixture over a saucepan of boiling water or the base of a double boiler after the chocolate is melted and well mixed (make sure the bottom of the bowl does not touch the water). Before serving, let it cool for a while. In a large mixing basin, whisk the egg yolks with the remaining superfine sugar until they are light in color, thick, and creamy. Whisk the cornstarch, brown sugar, and milk until smooth in another basin. Pour into a saucepan and cook for 5 minutes over medium heat, stirring regularly, or until thickened. Before going into the chocolate mixture, let everything cool a little. In a sizable, spotless mixing bowl, whisk the egg whites until stiff peaks form using clean mixer beaters. The chocolate mixture should be poured into the soufflé dishes until it is approximately 14 inches (5 mm) below the rim. Gently fold it in with a broad metal spoon. When the soufflés have fully risen, place the plates on a baking sheet and bake for 20 to 25 minutes. They should be served immediately after being dusted with confectioners' sugar since they will sink if left to stand.

6.17 AMARETTI TIRAMISU

Ingredients

4 large eggs, separated

½ cup superfine sugar, plus more for the coffee (optional) 12 ounces reduced-fat cream cheese, at room temperature 1 cup strong brewed coffee

¼ cup Marsala or amaretto (optional) About 30 Amaretti

Chocolate Sauce

½ teaspoon instant coffee ⅔ cup confectioners' sugar

2 heaping tablespoons unsweetened cocoa powder, plus more for dusting

Instructions

In a broad bowl, beat the egg yolks and superfine sugar with a hand-held electric mixer until thick, creamy, and pale. Beat in the cream cheese for 3 to 4 minutes, or until it is creamy and well-combined. The mixer's beaters should be cleaned. Whisk the egg whites in a large, spotless mixing bowl until firm peaks form. Using a large metal spoon, gently fold the egg whites into the cream cheese mixture. Combine the coffee, sugar, and liqueur in a small bowl (if using). Coffee should be dipped into each Amaretti biscuit. One cookie and a few tablespoons of the cream cheese filling should be placed on each of the six glass dessert plates. The remaining cookies and filling should be added last, followed by a cream cheese layer. To make the chocolate sauce, dissolve the instant coffee in two to three tablespoons of hot water. Sift the confectioners' sugar and cocoa together in a small mixing basin. Add the coffee mixture and whisk until smooth. Sprinkle some cocoa powder on top after drizzling the chocolate sauce over the tiramisu. Cover and refrigerate for at least two hours, preferable overnight, before serving.

6.18 IRISH CREAM DELIGHTS

Ingredients

½ cup light cream

½ cup packed light brown sugar

2 cups milk, lactose-free milk, or suitable plant-based milk ½ cup Irish cream liqueur, such as Baileys

¼ cup cornstarch

Shaved chocolate, for serving

Instructions

13/4 cup (435 ml) of the milk, cream, and brown sugar should all be combined in a medium pot. The mixture should be simmered until almost boiling. Mix thoroughly after adding the alcohol. The remaining 14 cups (60 ml) of milk should be combined with the cornstarch to create a smooth paste. Stirring regularly will help prevent lumps as you gradually add the mixture to the warm cream mixture. After about 5 minutes of simmering over medium heat, the sauce will have thickened. (Avoid letting it boil.) The pudding should be placed in six 4-ounce (125-ml) ramekins. Before wrapping with plastic wrap and chilling for 3 to 4 hours, or until set, let the mixture cool fully. Add shaved chocolate as a garnish right before serving.

6.19 BERRY AND CHOCOLATE FUDGE SUNDAES

Ingredients

Chocolate Fudge Sauce

3 tablespoons unsalted butter

½ cup packed light brown sugar ½ cup light cream

2 heaping tablespoons unsweetened cocoa powder

¼ cup good-quality dark chocolate buttons or chips

1-⅓ cups blueberries, 1-⅔ cups raspberries

3-⅓ cups strawberries, hulled, halved if large

4 cups gluten-free, lactose-free vanilla ice cream

Instructions

To make the chocolate fudge sauce, melt the butter in a little pot over low heat. Up to the chocolate has melted and the sauce is smooth, stir in the dark chocolate, brown sugar, milk, cocoa, and cocoa powder. After removing from the heat, let cooling to reach room temperature. The berries should be combined in a bowl. Place a large amount of chocolate fudge sauce on top of the berries before scooping the ice cream into serving cups or bowls.

6.20 WARM LEMON TAPIOCA PUDDING

Ingredients

4 lemons

4 cups low-fat milk, lactose-free milk, or suitable plant-based milk ½ cup pearl tapioca or sago

⅓ cup superfine sugar

Instructions

Using a vegetable peeler, cut the zest of all four lemons into 34-inch (2-cm) strips. Juicing the lemons yields 1/2 cup of lemon juice. The milk and lemon zest should be combined in a medium saucepan and heated over high heat until boiling. Turn the heat down to lower and cook the food for an additional two minutes. Lemon zest should be removed and discarded. The milk and tapioca should be well mixed after stirring. The tapioca should simmer for 20 to 25 minutes, stirring often, to transform it into translucent, jelly-like balls. Cut the heat off. Mix thoroughly after adding the sugar and lemon juice to the six glass dessert plates. Serve immediately.

6.21 WHITE CHOCOLATE–MINT POTS

Ingredients

2 cups milk, lactose-free milk, or suitable plant-based milk 1/4 cup light cream

1/2 cup superfine sugar

¼ teaspoon peppermint extract (more to taste) 3 or
4 drops green food coloring

4 ounces white chocolate chips, plus more for
decorating ¼ cup cornstarch

Mint leaves

Instructions

In a little saucepan over medium heat, bring 13/4
cup (185 ml) of milk, cream, sugar, peppermint
flavoring, and food coloring to a simmer (do not let
it boil). The white chocolate chips should be well
melted before being added. The remaining 14 cups
(60 ml) of milk should be combined with the
cornstarch to create a smooth paste. Stirring
regularly to prevent lumps, gradually add the white
chocolate mixture to the white chocolate mixture.
Cook for five minutes while stirring often, or until
the sauce has thickened. The ingredients should be
put into four 7-ounce (200 ml) ramekins. Before

placing in the refrigerator for 3 to 4 hours, or until hard, let the food cool fully at room temperature. Add fresh mint leaves and more white chocolate chips as a garnish just before serving.

6.22 CAPPUCCINO AND VANILLA BEAN MOUSSE DUO

Ingredients

Nonstick cooking spray

8 ounces good-quality white chocolate, broken into pieces 2/3 cup light cream

1 heaping tablespoon unflavored gelatin powder 4 large eggs, separated, at room temperature

1 cup light whipping cream 1/4 cup superfine sugar

1 teaspoon vanilla bean paste or 1 to 2 teaspoons vanilla extract 2 teaspoons instant coffee

Edible organic flowers (optional)

Instructions

Use nonstick cooking spray to coat six 5-ounce (150 ml) cups or ramekins. Mix the chocolate and light cream in a heatproof bowl or on the top of a double boiler. Stir over a pan of simmering water or the base of a double boiler until melted and well mixed (make sure the bottom of the bowl does not touch the water). Give cooling for 15 to 20 minutes. Pour 12 cups (125 ml) of cool water into a small heatproof bowl, then stir in the gelatin with a fork. The gelatin should soften after 5 minutes of being set aside. Hot water should be added to a giant bowl halfway, the gelatin bowl added, and the mixture continually whisked until the gelatin was completely dissolved. Egg yolks are added one at a time after the gelatin has been incorporated into the cooled chocolate mixture. Transferring half of the chocolate mixture to a different basin is necessary. Whipping cream and sugar should be whisked together in a clean mixing bowl using a handheld electric mixer until the liquid is thick and the sugar has completely dissolved. Put one-half of the whipped cream in a smaller bowl. The mixer's beaters should be cleaned. Whisk the egg whites in a large, spotless mixing bowl until firm peaks form. Add the vanilla essence to one of the bowls holding the chocolate mixture. With a large metal spoon, thoroughly incorporate this into one of the whipped cream dishes. Finally, carefully fold in half of the beaten egg whites. Fill the glasses with the mixture. For an hour, or until set, cover and refrigerate. The remaining bowls should be given time to warm up. After an hour, combine the leftover chocolate mixture with the coffee dissolved in 2 teaspoons of hot water. Fold the rest of it. Add the whipped cream to this, then carefully fold the remaining egg whites. Pour onto the glasses' vanilla layer. For two hours, or until set, cover, and refrigerate. If wanted, add a floral garnish right before serving.

6.23 CINNAMON PANNA COTTA WITH PUREED BANANA

Ingredients

Nonstick cooking spray 12/3 cups light cream

1/2 cup milk, lactose-free milk, or suitable plant-based milk 1/2 cup superfine sugar

1 teaspoon ground cinnamon 1 teaspoon vanilla extract

21/4 teaspoons unflavored gelatin powder Ice cubes

2 ripe bananas, peeled

2 teaspoons light brown sugar

Instructions

Spray four 4-ounce (125-ml) dariole molds, custard cups, or tall ramekins with cooking spray. Combine the cream, milk, superfine sugar, cinnamon, and vanilla in a medium saucepan over low heat. Cook, stirring regularly and taking care not to let it boil for 20 minutes or until the mixture is thick enough to coat the back of a spoon. Remove the pan from the heat and place it in a medium heatproof bowl. One tablespoon of cold water and the gelatin in a small heatproof dish, combined with a fork. Allow 5 minutes or until the gelatin begins to gel. Fill a giant bowl partly with boiling water, add the gelatin bowl, and stir until thoroughly dissolved. Using a whisk, incorporate the cream mixture. Half-fill a large mixing bowl with ice cubes. Place the cream mixture in the bowl on the ice for about 10 minutes, whisking every few minutes. The mixture will thicken as it cools. Once it has thickened enough to coat the back of a spoon, carefully pour it into the molds. Refrigerate, covered, for 2 to 3 hours, or until set. Mash the bananas and brown sugar together with a fork in a mixing bowl until smooth and well combined. Dip each mold for a few seconds in hot water before turning it out onto plates to serve. Fill a piping bag with the pureed banana and pipe it onto the dishes (or dollop it straight onto the panna cotta).

6.24 ORANGE-SCENTED PANNA COTTA

Ingredients

Nonstick cooking spray

Orange Topping

2 tablespoons plus 2 teaspoons fresh orange juice, strained 2 tablespoons plus 2 teaspoons boiling water

2 tablespoons plus 2 teaspoons sugar 1½ teaspoons unflavored gelatin powder 1-2/3 cups light cream

½ cup milk, lactose-free milk, or suitable plant-based milk ½ cup superfine sugar

3 to 4 heaping tablespoons finely grated orange zest

2 tablespoons plus 2 teaspoons fresh orange juice,

strained 2¼ teaspoons unflavored gelatin powder

Ice cubes

Orange segments, for serving

Instructions

Cooking Spray four 4-ounce (125-ml) dariole molds, custard cups, or tall ramekins with cooking spray. Combine all of the topping ingredients in a small heatproof dish. Place the bowl over a larger basin of hot water and whisk until the gelatin is completely dissolved. Place a quarter of the orange topping in each cup. Place in the refrigerator for 1-2 hours, or until completely set. Combine the cream, milk, superfine sugar, orange zest, and orange juice in a medium saucepan over low heat. Cook, stirring periodically, for 20 minutes, or until the sauce has thickened enough to coat the back of a spoon. Place the pan in a medium heatproof basin after turning off the heat. With a fork, combine the gelatin in a small heatproof basin with 1 tablespoon cold water. Allow 5 minutes, or until the gelatin begins to gel. Fill a larger bowl partly with boiling water, add the gelatin bowl, and stir until thoroughly dissolved. Using a whisk, incorporate the cream mixture. Half-fill a second large basin with ice cubes. Place the cream mixture in the bowl on the ice for about 10 minutes, whisking every few minutes. The mixture will thicken as it cools. Once it has thickened enough to coat the back of a spoon, carefully pour it over the orange topping in the molds. Refrigerate, covered, for 2 to 3 hours, or until set. Dip the mold for a few seconds in hot water before turning it out onto plates to serve. Garnish with fresh orange segments.

6.25 MAPLE SYRUP BAVARIAN CREAM WITH QUICK PECAN BRITTLE

Ingredients

Nonstick cooking spray

3 large egg yolks, at room temperature ½ cup superfine sugar

½ cup maple syrup

½ cup low-fat milk, lactose-free milk, or suitable plant-based milk 1 heaping tablespoon unflavored gelatin powder

Ice cubes

1 cup light whipping cream

Quick Pecan Brittle

1¾ ounces gluten-free butterscotch candies ½ cup pecans, coarsely crushed

Instructions

Cooking spray six 4-ounce dariole molds, custard cups, or tall ramekins. In a medium mixing bowl, combine the egg yolks and sugar and beat with a handheld electric mixer for 2 - 3 minutes, or until thick and pale. In a medium saucepan over low heat, combine the maple syrup and milk. Whisk in the egg mixture and whisk with a wooden spoon for 5 minutes over very low heat, or up to thick enough to coat the back of a spoon. Don't let it get too hot. Removing from heat and transfer to a medium heatproof bowl. In a small heatproof dish, mix together 3 tablespoons cold water and the gelatin with a fork. Approve it to sit for 5 minutes, or until the gelatin begins to gel. Fill a bigger bowl halfway with hot water, place the gelatin-containing bowl in it, and continually whisk until the gelatin is completely dissolved. Until smooth, whisk the gelatin into the maple mixture. Make a big basin of ice cubes. Place the bowl with the maple mixture on the ice for about 10 minutes, whisking every few minutes. As it cools, the mixture will thicken. In a medium mixing basin, beat the cream with a handheld electric mixer until thick. With a broad metal spoon, fold in the cooled maple mixture until fully blended. Pour equally into the molds, then set on a baking sheet, wrap in plastic wrap, and leave in the refrigerator for 4-5 hours. To prepare the pecan brittle, in a small food processor or blender, mix the butterscotch and pecans and process until coarsely crushed (do not overprocess or you will end up with crumbs). To serve, immerse each mold briefly in hot water before turning it out onto plates. Immediately top with the pecan brittle.

6.26 LEMON TART

Ingredients

Nonstick cooking spray

Tart Crust

1 cup superfine white rice flour

1/2 cup cornstarch, plus more for kneading 1/2 cup soy flour

1 teaspoon xanthan gum or guar gum 1/4 cup superfine sugar

10 tablespoons cold unsalted butter, diced About 1/2 cup ice water

3/4 cup superfine sugar

One 8-ounce package mascarpone

1 heaping tablespoon finely grated lemon zest 2/3 cup fresh lemon juice

4 large eggs

Confectioners' sugar, for dusting

Instructions

Preheat the oven to 350 degrees F. (180 degrees Celsius). Grease a 9-inch (23-cm) fluted tart pan with cooking spray. To make the crust, sift together the rice flour, cornstarch, soy flour, and xanthan gum in a mixing dish. In a food processor, combine the superfine sugar and butter and pulse until the mixture resembles fine bread crumbs. While the motor is running, add the cold water a tablespoon at a time to make a soft dough. Dust your work surface lightly with cornstarch. Knead the dough up to it is smooth on the work surface. After covering in plastic wrap, place in the refrigerator for 30 minutes, and roll out the dough to an 18-inch thickness between two pieces of parchment paper (2 to 3 mm). Place the crust in the pan and neaten the edges by trimming them. After lining the crust with parchment paper and filling it with pie weights or rice, bake for 10 minutes or until lightly golden. Take out the parchment and the consequences. Preheat the oven to 325 degrees Fahrenheit (160 degrees Celsius). To prepare the filling, whisk together the superfine sugar, mascarpone, lemon zest, and lemon juice in a medium mixing dish using a handheld electric mixer. One at a time, to add the eggs and thoroughly beat after each addition. Bake in the heated crust for 30 to 35 minutes or until the filling is set. Allow cooling completely in the pan. Dust with confectioners' sugar before serving.

6.27 CITRUS RICE TART WITH RASPBERRY SAUCE

Ingredients

Nonstick cooking spray

1 cup medium-grain white rice 1/4 cup sugar

1/3 cup cornstarch 3 large eggs

1/2 cup light cream

1/2 teaspoon vanilla extract Grated zest of 1 orange

3/4 cup fresh orange juice Grated zest of 1 lemon

RASPBERRY SAUCE

One 15-ounce can raspberry in syrup, drained, reserving the juice. 1/4 cup raspberry juice (from the can)

1 heaping tablespoon confectioners' sugar

Instructions

Set the oven temperature to 325 degrees Fahrenheit (160 degrees Celsius). Grease a 9-inch (23-cm) fluted tart or pie pan with cooking spray. Bring 612 cups (1.5 liters) of water to a boil in a big pot. Add the rice and sugar if necessary, and cook for 12 minutes, stirring occasionally, or until the rice is tender. Drain and run a cold water rinse to chill. Mix the cornstarch, eggs, cream, vanilla, orange and lemon zests, as well as their juices, in a medium mixing dish. Well incorporate the rice. Bake the tart pan for 35 to 40 minutes, or until the filling is barely set. After to taking it out of the oven, put it in the refrigerator for two to three hours until it reaches room temperature. Take the food out of the fridge 30 minutes before serving. If the bottom of your pan is removable, take off the outside rim. To prepare the raspberry sauce, mix all the ingredients in a blender or food processor. Serve the tart with a drizzle.

6.28 LEMON TARTLETS

Ingredients

Nonstick cooking spray

Lemon Filling

½ cup cornstarch 1¼ cups water

Grated zest of 2 lemons ¾ cup fresh lemon juice

4 tablespoons unsalted butter, cut into cubes, at room temperature ⅔ cup sugar

2 large egg yolks

1 batch Tart Crust dough, chilled

Gluten-free, lactose-free ice cream, for serving

Instructions

Set the oven temperature to 325 degrees Fahrenheit (170 degrees Celsius). Grease a 12-cup muffin pan or twelve tartlet pans with cooking spray. In a little saucepan, combine the cornstarch with 1 tablespoon of water and stir until smooth to make the filling. To ensure there are no lumps before add the remaining water, followed by the butter, sugar, lemon juice, and zest. Continue cooking while stirring regularly for 3 to 5 minutes, or until the sauce has thickened. After removing from the heat, allow it cool for ten minutes. The egg yolks should be whisked together in a separate basin. Pour into a bowl, cover, and refrigerate up to very cold. Layout the chilled dough to a thickness of 18 inches between two sheets of parchment paper in the interim (2 to 3 mm). Cut out twelve circles with a pastry cutter so they will fit the pan or cups. To clean up the sides of the pan or cups, trim them. Bake for 12 to 15 minutes, or until golden brown, in a 350°F oven. Allow wire rack to cool fully. With ice cream on the side, fill the tartlet crusts with the chilled lemon filling.

6.29 CINNAMON AND CHESTNUT FLAN

Ingredients

Nonstick cooking spray

1 batch Tart Crust dough chilled ¾ cup superfine sugar

2 tablespoons ground cinnamon

One 14-ounce can fat-free sweetened condensed milk

One 8-ounce package mascarpone or reduced-fat cream cheese, at room temperature 1½ cups chestnut meal

4 large eggs

Confectioners' sugar, for dusting

Gluten-free, lactose-free ice cream, for serving

Instructions

Turn the oven's temperature up to 350 degrees (170 degrees Celsius). Grease a 9-inch (23-cm) fluted quiche pan with cooking spray. The chilled dough should be rolled out to a thickness of about 18 inches between two pieces of parchment paper (2 to 3 mm). Trim the crust's edges, then place it in the flan dish. After lining the crust with parchment paper and stuffing it with pie weights or rice, bake for 10 minutes, or until lightly browned.Transfer the baking sheet from the oven and reduce the temperature to 325°F (160°C). Remove the parchment and weights. While waiting, prepare the filling by pulsing the eggs, mascarpone, condensed milk, cinnamon, and chestnut meal in a food processor or blender up to well blended. The filling should be poured into the hot crust. In a 350°F oven, bake for 50 to 60 minutes, or until the food is firm. Before serving, remove from the pan and leave to completely cool. Serve topped with confectioners' sugar and ice cream.

6.30 LEMON CHEESECAKE

Ingredients

9 ounces gluten-free vanilla cookies, crushed (about 2½ cups) 4 tablespoons unsalted butter, melted

Cheesecake Filling

1 heaping tablespoon unflavored gelatin powder

One 8-ounce package of reduced-fat cream cheese, at room temperature ¾ cup superfine sugar

2 tablespoons plus 2 teaspoons fresh lemon juice 1 to 2 heaping tablespoons grated lemon zest 1⅓ cups light whipping cream

Lemon Topping

1½ teaspoons unflavored gelatin powder

3 tablespoons unsalted butter, cut into cubes, at room temperature ½ cup superfine sugar

1 large egg yolk, lightly beaten 1 teaspoon grated lemon zest

2 tablespoons plus 2 teaspoons fresh lemon juice

Instructions

The crushed cookies and melted butter should be combined in a medium mixing bowl.

Press evenly into the bottom of an 8-inch (20-cm) springform pan. While you work on the filling, refrigerate the topping and filling. To make the filling, put the gelatin in a small heatproof bowl and stir in 12 cups (125 ml) of cold water. Give it five minutes to settle or until the gelatin starts to gel. Hot water should be added to a giant mixing bowl halfway, the gelatin bowl added, and the mixture continually whisked until the gelatin was completely dissolved. Cream cheese, sugar, lemon juice, lemon zest, and dissolved gelatin should be combined in a food processor or blender and blended for one to two minutes until creamy. Use a handheld electric mixer to whisk the cream in a medium mixing bowl until it thickens. Use a large metal spoon, fold the whipped cream into the cream cheese mixture.Add the filling to the cookie shell. Three hours or until stiff, cover, and chill. To make the topping, combine the gelatin with a fork in a small heatproof bowl containing 1/2 cup (125 ml) of cold water. Give it five minutes to settle or until the gelatin starts to gel. Hot water should be added to a giant bowl halfway, the gelatin bowl added, and the mixture continually whisked until the gelatin was completely dissolved. The dissolved gelatin, butter, sugar, egg yolk, lemon juice, and zest should all be combined in a small pot. Over low heat, stir for around 15 minutes or until the sauce is sufficiently thick to coat the back of a spoon. Before serving, let the food cool to room temperature. Spread the topping evenly over the filling by placing the cheesecake back in the refrigerator for at least 3 hours or until it is hard.

6.31 BAKED BLUEBERRY CHEESECAKES

Ingredients

7 ounces gluten-free vanilla cookies, crushed (about 2 cups) 4 tablespoons unsalted butter, melted

2 cups fresh or frozen blueberries

Two 8-ounce packages of reduced-fat cream cheese at room temperature One 14-ounce can fat-free sweetened condensed milk

2 teaspoons vanilla extract ½ cup light whipping cream 2 large eggs, ¼ cup (35 g) cornstarch

Instructions

Set the oven's temperature to 325°F (160°C). Melted butter should be combined with the broken cookies before being pressed into the bottom of nine 4-inch (10-cm) springform pans. Over the cookie crusts, distribute the blueberries equally. In a food processor or blender, mash the cream cheese, condensed milk, vanilla, cream, eggs, and cornstarch until smooth. Over the crusts, pour the batter. Bake for 15 - 20 minutes, or until firm to the touch and gently brown. Allow to entirely cool in the pans before covering and chilling for three hours before serving.

6.32 CHOCOLATE TART

Ingredients

Nonstick cooking spray

7 ounces gluten-free chocolate cookies, crushed (about 2 cups) 5 tablespoons unsalted butter, melted

Chocolate Filling

8 ounces good-quality dark chocolate, broken into piecesio tablespoons unsalted butter, cut into cubes, at room temperature 3/4 cup superfine sugar

2 teaspoons vanilla extract

1/4 cup coffee liqueur (optional) 5 large eggs, at room temperature

Unsweetened cocoa powder for dusting

Gluten-free, lactose-free, ice cream, for serving

Instructions

Turn the oven's temperature up to 300 degrees (150 degrees Celsius). Grease a 9-inch (23-cm) fluted tart pan with cooking spray. The crushed cookies and melted butter should be combined in a medium mixing bowl. Press evenly in the tart pan's bottom. Keep the filling chilled while you are preparing it. To making the filling, put the chocolate in a small heat-resistant bowl or the top of a double boiler. Set with the bottom of a double boiler or a pot of hot water nearby. Stir occasionally until the wax melts (make sure the bottom of the bowl does not contact the water). Before serving, allow for a little cooling. Using a handheld electric mixer to blend the butter, sugar, vanilla, coffee liqueur (if using), and 1 egg in a medium mixing bowl until they are light and fluffy. Add the melted chocolate and stir everything together thoroughly. Take it out of the equation. The mixer's beaters should be cleaned. The remaining eggs should be whisked in a sizable mixing bowl for 3 to 5 minutes, or until they have doubled in volume. The eggs and chocolate mixture should be combined entirely after 1 to 2 minutes of low-speed beating. The filling should be evenly distributed throughout the cookie dough. Bake for 45 to 50 minutes, or until hard. Remove from the oven, allow it cool to room temperature, and then chill for two to three hours. Serve with ice cream and generously sprinkled with cocoa powder.

6.33 PECAN AND MAPLE TARTS

Ingredients

Nonstick cooking spray

2 batches Tart Dough, chilled Filling

1 tablespoon unsalted butter, at room temperature

1/4 cup packed light brown sugar

1/2 teaspoon vanilla extract 1 large egg

1/4 cup maple syrup

1/2 cup pecans, roughly chopped Confectioners' sugar, for dusting (optional)

Instructions

Set the oven heat to 325 degrees Fahrenheit (170 degrees Celsius). Grease two 12-cup mini tartlet or mini muffin pans with cooking spray. A bake sheet should be lined with parchment paper. Between two pieces of parchment paper, roll out the chilled pastry dough to a thickness of approximately 18 inches (2 to 3 mm). Use a scalloped 1- to 112-inch (3- to 4-cm) pastry cutter to cut out 24 rounds of crust to suit the mini tartlet pans. Clean up the edges before placing in the cups. Using a cookie cutter in the form of a star, make 24 little stars (or any preferred form). Arrange the stars on the baking sheet. Bake the crusts and stars in a 350°F oven until they are golden (the crusts will take about 10 minutes, but the stars will only need 7 to 8 minutes). The pan should be taken out of the oven and set on a wire rack to cool. Turn the oven's temperature up to 350 degrees (180 degrees Celsius). Use a hand-held electric mixer to thoroughly blend the butter, brown sugar, and vanilla in a small mixing bowl. After mixing in the egg and maple syrup, stir in the chopped pecans. Equally distribute the mixture between the crusts and bake for 5 to 10 minutes, or until the filling is set (it should remain firm when given a gentle shake). Put a star on each tart while it's still warm. Cool in the pans for ten minutes before transferring to a wire rack to finish cooling. Dust with confectioners' sugar if preferred.

6.34 CARROT CAKE WITH CREAM CHEESE FROSTING

Ingredients

Nonstick cooking spray

⅓ cup superfine white rice flour ⅓ cup cornstarch

2 teaspoons gluten-free baking powder 1 teaspoon baking soda

1 teaspoon xanthan gum or guar gum

1 heaping tablespoon ground cinnamon 1 heaping tablespoon pumpkin pie spice 2 cups almond flour

1 cup packed light brown sugar 2 medium carrots, grated

⅓ cup walnuts, chopped 4 large eggs, separated

Cream Cheese Frosting

One 8-ounce package reduced-fat cream cheese 1 tablespoon plus 1 teaspoon fresh lemon juice ½ cup confectioners' sugar

Instructions

The oven's setting should be 325 degrees Fahrenheit (160 degrees Celsius). Cooking Spray and line a loaf pan that measures 812 x 412 inches (22 x 11.5 cm) with parchment paper, leaving an overhang on the two long edges to help lift the cake out later. Sift the rice flour, cornstarch, baking powder, baking soda, xanthan gum, cinnamon, and pumpkin pie spice together three times in a large mixing basin (or whisk in the bowl until well combined). In a mixing dish, combine the almond flour, brown sugar, carrots, walnuts, and egg yolks. I use a handheld electric mixer to whisk the egg whites in a medium mixing basin until stiff peaks form. A big metal spoon should be used to carefully mix the egg whites into the carrot batter. After filling the pan halfway, bake for 45 to 50 minutes, or until the batter feels firm to the touch (a toothpick inserted into the center should come out clean). Before transferring the dish to a wire rack to finish cooling, let it rest in the pan for 10 minutes. The cream cheese frosting is made by whipping cream cheese, lemon juice, and confectioners' sugar. Once the cake has cooled, spread the icing over the top and serve.

6.35 LAYERED TAHITIAN LIME CHEESECAKE

Ingredients

9 ounces gluten-free vanilla cookies, crushed

4 tablespoons butter, melted

2 tablespoons unflavored gelatin powder

Two 8-ounce packages of reduced-fat cream cheese at room temperature One 14-ounce can fat-free sweetened condensed milk

1/3 cup coconut liqueur

3 tablespoons plus 1 teaspoon fresh lime juice Finely grated zest of 1 lime

1 to 2 drops of green food coloring

Instructions

In a medium dish, combine the butter that has been melted with the crumbled cookies. A 9-inch (23 cm) springform pan should have an equal layer of crust on the bottom. While you make the topping, place in the fridge. Gelatin should be dissolved in 12 cup (125 ml) of cold water before being added to a small heatproof dish. Wait until the gelatin starts to gel, about 5 minutes. Set the bowl containing the gelatin in a bigger basin filled with boiling water, and stir continuously until the gelatin has completely dissolved. In a food processor or blender, combining the cream cheese, condensed milk, and dissolved gelatin. Process for one minute, or until smooth. There should be roughly 2 cups of mixture left after you pour half of it into a clean basin (500 ml). Mix in the coconut liqueur after adding it to the bowl. Pour over the cookie crust, then 10 minutes of freezing. The remaining batter in the food processor should be mixed well when you add the lime juice, lime zest, and food coloring. The cheesecake should be just about set when taken out of the freezer. Pour the lime mixture over the coconut layer, and then place the dish in the refrigerator for two to three hours to thoroughly set.

6.36 ORANGE AND POPPY SEED CAKE

Ingredients

Nonstick cooking spray 2 oranges

1¼ cups almond flour

1 teaspoon gluten-free baking powder ½ cup (65 g) superfine white rice flour 2 tablespoons poppy seeds

5 large eggs 1¼ cups sugar

Instructions

Set the oven's temperature to 325°F (170°C). A 9-inch (23 cm) springform pan should be greased with cooking spray and lined with a circle of parchment paper. The oranges should be covered and boiled in a medium saucepan for 20 minutes. Drain. For a smooth paste, purée the softened oranges (seeds, pith, and all!) in a food processor or blender for 3 - 4 minutes. Before serving, allow cooling. Three times sift the rice flour, baking powder, and almond flour into a mixing basin (or whisk in the bowl until well combined). Mix thoroughly after adding the poppy seeds. Using a handheld electric mixer to whisk the eggs in a medium mixing bowl for 5 minutes or until thick and creamy. Add the sugar and stir everything together thoroughly. Using a large metal spoon, incorporate the orange paste into the egg mixture after mixing it into the dry ingredients. Bake for 50-60 minutes, or up to golden brown and firm to the touch, after filling the pan halfway with batter (a toothpick inserted into the center should come out clean).

After fifteen minutes of cooling in the pan, remove the outer ring and let the cake cool on a wire rack.

6.37 RICH WHITE CHOCOLATE CAKE

Ingredients

Nonstick cooking spray

15 tablespoons unsalted butter, cut into cubes

7 ounces good-quality white chocolate, broken into pieces 2¼ cups packed light brown sugar

¾ cup soy flour

¾ cup tapioca flour

1 cup superfine white rice flour ½ cup cornstarch

2 teaspoons xanthan gum or guar gum 1 teaspoon baking soda

1 teaspoon gluten-free baking powder 2 teaspoons vanilla extract

2 large eggs

Confectioners' sugar, for dusting

Instructions

Turn the oven's temperature up to 300 degrees (150 degrees Celsius). Grease a 9-inch (23-cm) springform pan with cooking spray. Combine the butter, white chocolate, brown sugar, and 112 cups (375 ml) of boiling water in a medium heatproof dish or the top of a double boiler. Placing the dish over a pot of boiling water or the bottom of a double boiler to melt the chocolate and butter and ensure that everything is completely mixed . Allow food to cool to room temperature before serving. Sift the soy flour, tapioca flour, rice flour, cornstarch, xanthan gum, baking soda, and baking powder three times in a medium mixing bowl (or whisk in the bowl until well combined). Whip the cooled white chocolate mixture, vanilla, and eggs until smooth using a hand-held electric mixer. After putting the mixture into the pan, bake for 45 minutes. Bake for a further 15 to 30 minutes, or until firm, covered with foil. After 15 minutes of cool in the pan, remove the outer ring and let the cake cool completely on a wire rack. Dust with confectioners' sugar just before serving.

6.38 FLOURLESS CHOCOLATE CAKE

Ingredients

Nonstick cooking spray

1/3 cup unsweetened cocoa powder, plus more for dusting

10 tablespoons unsalted butter, cut into cubes, at room temperature 5 ounces good-quality dark chocolate, broken into pieces

1¼ cups packed light brown sugar 1¼ cups almond flour

4 large eggs, separated

Gluten-free, lactose-free ice cream, for serving (optional)

Instructions

Turn the oven's temperature up to 300 degrees (150 degrees Celsius). Cooking spray should be used to line a 9-inch (23-cm) springform pan with parchment paper. The cocoa, butter, dark chocolate, and 13 cups (80 ml) water should all be placed in a medium saucepan over low heat and whisked until smooth. Add the egg yolks, brown sugar, and almond flour after turning off the heat in the pan. In a large mixing bowl, let cooling to room temperature. Using a clean mixing bowl and a handheld electric mixer, beat the egg whites until soft peaks form. Gently incorporate the egg whites into the cooled chocolate mixture in two batches. Pour the batter into the prepared springform pan and bake for 55 to 65 minutes, until the middle is firm when lightly touched. Cooling for twenty minutes in the pan before removing the outer ring and turning it onto a wire rack to cool fully. If desired, top with more chocolate and serve with ice cream.

6.39 MOIST CHOCOLATE CAKE

Ingredients

Nonstick cooking spray

1 cup plus 2 tablespoons superfine white rice flour

1/2 cup cornstarch

1/2 cup potato flour

2/3 cup unsweetened cocoa powder

2 teaspoons gluten-free baking powder 1 teaspoon baking soda

1 teaspoon xanthan gum or guar gum 2 large eggs

1½ cups superfine sugar

3 tablespoons unsalted butter, melted

¾ cup gluten-free, low-fat vanilla yogurt

⅔ cup low-fat milk, lactose-free milk, or suitable plant-based milk

Chocolate Frosting

1½ cups confectioners' sugar

2 to 3 heaping tablespoons unsweetened cocoa powder 7 tablespoons unsalted butter, at room temperature

¼ cup low-fat milk, lactose-free milk, or suitable plant-based milk

Instructions

The oven's setting should be 325 degrees Fahrenheit (170 degrees Celsius). Using cooking spray, line a 9-

inch (23-cm) springform pan with a circle of parchment paper. Sift the rice flour, cornstarch, potato flour, cocoa, baking powder, baking soda, and xanthan gum three times in a large mixing basin (or whisk in the bowl until well combined). The eggs and fine sugar should be whisked together in a medium mixing dish until foamy and thick. Yogurt, milk, and melted butter are all added while stirring continuously. With a wooden spoon, combine the addition with the dry ingredients for 2 to 3 minutes, or until all lumps are gone. Bake for 45 - 55 minutes, or until the batter feels firm to the touch, after filling the pan halfway (a toothpick inserted in the center should come out clean). Before removing the outer ring and transferring to a wire rack to finish cooling, let the food cool for 10 minutes in the pan. To create the chocolate frosting, sift the confectioners' sugar and cocoa into a mixing bowl. Add the butter and milk and stir everything together thoroughly. Spread the mixture evenly over the cooled cake using a spatula.

6.40 HAZELNUT–SOUR CREAM CAKE WITH BLUEBERRY JAM

Ingredients

Nonstick cooking spray

13 tablespoons unsalted butter, cut into cubes at room temperature 1½ cups superfine sugar

2 teaspoons vanilla extract 3 large eggs

¾ cup superfine white rice flour ⅓ cup soy flour

¼ cup cornstarch

1 teaspoon ground cinnamon 1 teaspoon baking soda

2 teaspoons gluten-free baking powder 1 teaspoon xanthan gum or guar gum 1 cup hazelnut flour

1 cup light sour cream

Cream Cheese Filling

4 ounces reduced-fat cream cheese, at room temperature ½ cup hazelnut flour

1 teaspoon ground cinnamon ⅔ cup confectioners' sugar

1 tablespoon plus 1 teaspoon fresh lemon juice ½ cup blueberry jam, plus more for garnish

Instructions

Turn the oven's temperature up to 350 degrees (180 degrees Celsius). Spray with cooking spray and line with circles of parchment paper two 8-inch (22-cm) cake pans. Use a handheld electric mixer to combine the butter, superfine sugar, and vanilla in a large mixing bowl and beat up to thick, creamy, and pale. One at a time, adding the eggs, beating thoroughly after each addition.Sift the rice flour, soy flour, cornstarch, cinnamon, baking soda, baking powder, and xanthan gum three times in a medium mixing bowl (or whisk in the bowl until well combined). Incorporate the hazelnut flour well. Using a large metal spoon, slowly fold the dry ingredients into the butter mixture in two parts, alternating with the sour cream. In an even layer, pour the batter into the pans. 35–40 minutes of baking time, or until a toothpick inserted in the center of the cake comes out clean. Cool in the pans for ten minutes before transferring to a wire rack to finish cooling. All of the cream cheese filling's components should be combined and thoroughly stirred in a medium mixing basin. The jam should be poured over one of the cake layers, followed by about half of the cream cheese filling. The leftover cream cheese mixture should be spread on top of the second layer of cake. Add a layer of blueberry jam as a garnish.

6.41 BROWNIE BATTER BOWLS

Ingredients

¼ cup butter softened, plus more for greasing ramekins 1 tablespoon unsweetened cocoa powder

½ cup sugar

1 tablespoon cornstarch

6 ounces semi-sweet chocolate, chopped 1 teaspoon vanilla extract

2 large eggs, lightly beaten

6 tablespoons vanilla lactose-free ice cream 2 tablespoons pomegranate seeds

Instructions

Set the oven to 300 degrees Fahrenheit. Six 4- to 5-ounce ramekins should be lightly buttered on the bottom and halfway up the sides before being dusted with cocoa powder. Arrange the ramekins on a baking sheet. In a small mixing dish, combine the sugar and cornstarch. Putting butter and chocolate in a medium microwave-safe dish.Microwave on high for 1 minute, then stir. Rep at 20- to 30-second intervals until the chocolate and butter have melted fully. Combine the melted chocolate, sugar mixture, and vanilla extract in a mixing bowl. One at a time, adding the eggs, beating well with a wooden spoon after each addition. Preheat the oven to 350°F and divide the batter among the ramekins. Bake for 30 minutes, or until the brownie is puffy and cracked around the sides of each ramekin but the middle is still soft. Allow it to cool on a cake rack for 15 minutes before serving with a scoop of ice cream and a few pomegranate seeds.

6.42 CHOCOLATE -DIPPED ALMOND BISCOTTI

Ingredients

½ cup salted butter, softened 1 cup sugar

2 large eggs

2 tablespoons water

1 tablespoon almond extract 1 tablespoon vanilla extract ½ cup almond flour

¾ cup/80 grams sorghum flour

1¾ cups/190 grams Authentic Foods Superfine Brown Rice Flour 6 tablespoons tapioca starch

3 tablespoons cornstarch

3 tablespoons arrowroot powder 2 tablespoons ground chia seeds 2 teaspoons baking powder

½ cup almond slices

1 cup semi-sweet chocolate chips 2 teaspoons coconut oil

Instructions

Set the oven's temperature to 325 degrees. Prepare by preparing two large baking pans with foil. In a large mixing bowl, stir the butter and sugar together using a wooden spoon. Beat ferociously after each addition of an egg, one at a time. Add the water along with the almond and vanilla extracts. In a medium mix bowl, combine the flours, tapioca starch, cornstarch, and arrowroot powder. Stir in the chia seeds and baking powder until well incorporated. At each addition, add about a quarter of this mixture, thoroughly combining between branches. If additional rice flour is required, add one tablespoon at a time until the dough is firm and keeps its shape. Mix thoroughly after adding the almonds. Make a 3-inch-wide loaf of dough about an inch thick on each baking sheet by dividing the dough in half. Smooth the tops of the loaves using damp fingertips. After the first 20 minutes, rotate the baking pans in the oven and bake for 45 to 50 minutes until golden and firm to the touch. Cold for five minutes on the baking sheets, then tightly wrap in foil and place in an excellent place to cool. Set the oven's temperature to 300 degrees. Unwrap one loaf, then set it on a cutting board. Cut the bread into 34-inch-thick slices on the diagonal using a broad serrated knife and a moderate sawing motion. Take care and support when handling the bread. Then, carefully place the pieces in a single layer on a baking sheet that has been greased. Repeat the process with a different baking sheet and the second loaf, saving any crumbs that appear. Bake for 40 to 50 minutes until everything is evenly golden brown. After turning off the oven and opening the door, let the cookies finish cooling in the cooling oven. Chocolate chips and coconut oil should be placed in a small glass cup or plate and microwaved on high for 30 seconds, stirring after each interval, until smooth and melted. Each biscotti should be dipped in chocolate and placed on parchment or wax paper. Sprinkle any remaining crumbs on top of the warm chocolate. Once the chocolate has hardened, store the biscotti in an airtight container until ready to serve.

6.43 LEMON -PECAN BARS

Ingredients

⅓ cup salted butter ⅔ cup oat flour

⅔ cup finely ground pecan flour 4 large eggs

1 ⅓ cups granulated sugar 1 teaspoon vanilla extract

1 teaspoon almond extract ⅓ cup fresh lemon juice

1 tablespoon cornstarch

1½ teaspoons baking powder Pinch of salt

Confectioners' sugar (optional)

Instructions

350 degrees Fahrenheit should be the oven's temperature setting. In a medium microwave-safe bowl, warm the butter for 15 seconds on high to gradually soften it. With a wooden spoon, mix the flour, one egg, 13 cups of granulated sugar, vanilla,

and almond extracts until a soft dough forms. In a 9-inch square baking pan, press the dough. On a rack in the bottom third of the oven, bake for 30 minutes, or up to firm to the touch and golden brown around the edges.Set the oven's temperature to 350 degrees Fahrenheit. Beat the remaining 1 cup sugar, lemon juice, cornstarch, baking powder, three eggs, and salt in a medium bowl for 3 minutes on medium-high speed with an electric mixer. Pour the mixture over and put the baking dish back in the oven. Bake for 20 minutes on the same rack, then reduce the heat to 300°F and bake for 10 minutes until the custard is bubbly and light golden brown. The dish shouldn't seem runny below when it is inverted. Before cutting the lemon bars into squares, let them cool in the pan.

If preferred, top with confectioners' sugar right before serving. Refrigerate leftovers after placing them in an airtight container.

6.44 RASPBERRY-LIME ICE POPS

Ingredients

1½ cups cold water 10 tablespoons sugar

4 tablespoons fresh lime juice (from 2 limes)

1½ cups mashed fresh (about 3 cups) or frozen-thawed (12 ounces) raspberries

10 wooden pop sticks

Instructions

In a medium saucepan over medium temperature, bring the water and sugar to a boil while stirring c\ontinuously until the sugar is dissolved. Add the lime juice and raspberries after removing it from the heat. Fill the molds with the mixture using a kitchen funnel. Tap the molds frequently on the counter to help the mixture settle in the molds. Dip a pop stick into each mold a few times to push any air bubbles to the top.For one hour, put the molds in the freezer. 10 wooden ice pop sticks should each have one end placed in a glass of water that is 2 inches deep with cold water. Before placing the sticks inside the ice pop molds, dry them off with a towel. For at least another four hours, freeze. The freezing period may change based on the freezer's temperature. For about 30 seconds, submerge the ice-pop molds in very warm water before unmolding and serving. In sandwich bags, leftover pops may be frozen for many weeks.

6.45 FIVE-INGREDIENT PEANUT BUTTER COOKIES

Ingredients

1 large egg

1 cup peanut butter

¾ cup sugar, plus extra for forming cookies ¼ cup miniature semi-sweet chocolate chips ⅛ teaspoon sea salt or kosher salt flakes

Instructions

350 degrees Fahrenheit should be the oven's temperature setting. Stir the egg, peanut butter, and 34 cups sugar together thoroughly in a medium mixing bowl. then incorporate the chocolate chips. Roll the dough into twenty-eight 1-inch balls using your hands or a tiny cookie scoop, then place them on two ungreased cookie trays. To make a crisscross design, press the back of the fork into the dough of the first biscuit. Before spreading the tops of the cookies to a thickness of approximately 14 inches, dip the fork tines in some loose sugar. Add a little salt to the cookies to season them. Bake the cookies for 12 to 14 minutes, or until puffy in the middle and firm around the edges, in a 350°F preheated oven. Never overbake them, please. Before putting the cookies in an airtight container, allow the cookies to cool fully. \

6.46 VEGAN KHIR PUDDING

Ingredients

1 cup cashews, soaked in water for 4 hours, and drained 1 to 11/2 cups water

2 to 3 tablespoons maple syrup, or to taste Pinch of sea salt

1 to 2 teaspoons of cardamom, or to taste

1/2 cup cooked brown rice or whole-grain noodles (such as rice or buckwheat noodles of your choice)

Dash of saffron (optional)

1/4 cup slivered almonds (optional)

Instructions

Blend the cashews, water, maple syrup, cardamom, and salt to taste in a blender.

Cooked rice or noodles should be combined with cashew milk, saffron, almonds, and an additional drop of maple syrup, if desired.

6.47 COCONUT CURRANT COOKIES

Ingredients

1 egg

1/2 cup honey

1/4 teaspoon salt

1/2 cup almond flour

1 1 /2 cups shredded coconut 1 /2 cup chopped walnuts

1/2 cup currants

Instructions

350 degrees should be the prepared oven temperature. Salt, honey, and eggs should be combined in a blender or electric mixer. Almond flour should be added and well mixed. After adding the currants, walnuts, and coconut, thoroughly combine. Bake for 10 to 12 minutes after preheating the oven to 350

6.48 COCONUT BREAD

Ingredients

2/3 cups coconut flour 5 eggs

1 teaspoon organic vanilla 2 teaspoons cinnamon

1/2 teaspoon salt

1 tablespoon of gluten-free baking powder 1/4 cup plus 1 tablespoon honey

Instructions

Achieve a 330 degree oven temperature. 1 teaspoon of cinnamon, 14 cups of honey, salt, and baking powder should all be combined in a mixing bowl. Half of the batter should be placed in a prepared 9 x 5 inch loaf pan or an oiled silicone bread pan. The remaining honey and cinnamon should be sprinkled over the dough before baking for 45 to 50 minutes.

6.49 DATE SYRUP

Ingredients

20 to 25 honey or Medjool dates

1 cup filtered, spring, or alkaline water

Instructions

Pit the dates and place them in a basin with the water. Take a 3- to 4-hour soak. Dates and soaking water are blended in a blender until completely smooth.

6.50 ANGEL'S DECADENT WHIPPED CREAM

Ingredients

1 cup macadamia nuts, soaked in water for 4 hours, and drained 1/2 cup water

1 /2 cup Date Syrup or agave, or more to taste 1 teaspoon organic vanilla

1 tablespoon cold-pressed coconut oil

Instructions

In a blender, combine all the ingredients and process until they are smooth and creamy.

6.51 FROZEN FRUIT POPS

Ingredients

2 cups fresh mango 1 teaspoon lemon juice 1 teaspoon brown sugar or agave (optional) 1/2 cup water

Instructions

The fruit and lemon juice should be blended until smooth in a food processor. Taste it and, if necessary, add more brown sugar or agave nectar to make it sweeter. Place the mixture in large ice cube trays or miniature glasses and freeze until slushy (15 to 45 minutes, depending on cup size and the temperature of your freezer). Once the liquid has become slushy, insert the Popsicle sticks and freeze for up to two hours.

6.52 BANANA SMOOTHIE

Ingredients

3 bananas

1 1/2 cup lactose-free milk 1 teaspoon honey

1/3 cup ice cubes

Instructions

All the components should be smooth after being combined.

6.53 RASPBERRY SMOOTHIE

Ingredients

1 cup raspberries

1 1/2 cup lactose-free milk 1 teaspoon honey

1/3 cup ice cubes

Instructions

All of the components should be thoroughly blended.

6.54 NUTTY BREAKFAST SMOOTHIE

Ingredients:

2 bananas

2 cups spinach 1 cup water

1 tablespoon almond butter

Instructions:

Slice the spinach and bananas. Blend together all the ingredients. Blend until smooth, then savor.

6.55 SAFE AND SOOTHING SMOOTHIE

Ingredients:

1 small, ripe banana

1 cup strawberries, fresh or frozen

2 tablespoons hulled hemp seeds (no soaking required)

1 to 2 tablespoons pea powder protein (such as provided)

1 cup liquid (water, coconut juice, or half coconut juice and half coconut milk) Natural sweetener (such as agave, stevia, or Just Like Sugar) to taste (optional)

Instructions:

Banana, strawberries, hemp seeds, and pea powder are combined in a powerful blender or food processor. Blend in the liquid, being sure to thoroughly coat each ingredient. If necessary, taste the mixed mixture and adjust the sweetness (if desired). The mixture should be blended briefly one more time to include any sweetness.

6.56 BANANA AND GREENS DELIGHT SMOOTHIE

Ingredients:

1 banana, cut up

2 cups baby spinach, chopped

1 apple, cored, peeled, and cut up 1 pear, cored, peeled, and cut up 2 cups water

Instructions:

In a blender or with a strong hand blender, combine all the ingredients. After blending until smooth, serve.

6.57 LOVELY BONES JUICE

Ingredients:

2 apples, quartered 5 kale leaves

1 handful parsley (about 1/2 cup)

Juice of 1/4 of a lemon (about 1/16 cup) 1-inch ginger

1 celery stalk

Instructions:

Alternatively, you may puree the ingredients together in a blender, then purify the resulting liquid using a nut milk bag (for more information on this procedure, see the nearby sidebar 'Juicer or nut milk bag: That is the question'). To serve, pour the mixture into glasses.

6.58 GINGER LOVE!

Ingredients:

1/4 inch ginger

2 apples, quartered

Juice of 1/2 a lemon (about 1/8 cup)

Instructions:

Juice the ginger first, followed by the apple quarters, or chop, mix, then strain through a nut milk bag. Lemon juice should be squeezed on the dish.

6.59 PICK ME UP

Ingredients:

1 bunch cilantro (about 12 ounces) 3 apples, cored and quartered

1 medium cucumber, cut lengthwise 8 to 10 celery stalks Juice of 3 lemons (about 3/4 cup)

Instructions:

Apple, cucumber, celery, and cilantro may all be juiced, mixed, and then filtered through a nut milk bag.

Lemon juice should be squeezed on the dish.

6.60 SOAKING NUTS AND SEEDS

Ingredients:

1 cup nuts or seeds of your choice

1 /4 teaspoon of sea salt Water (enough to cover nuts/seeds)

Instructions:

The nuts or seeds should be rinsed in a fine sieve three times before being set aside. Combine the salt and water in a dish or other soaking container, then add the nuts or seeds. It is recommended to soak seeds for at least 4 hours and nuts for at least 8 hours. The nuts and seeds should be taken out of the soaking solution and properly rinsed under fresh water.

6.61 CASHEW MILK

Ingredients:

1 cup raw cashews, soaked (see Soaking Nuts and Seeds earlier in this chapter) 10 honey dates, soaked for 1 hour 2 cups water

Instructions:

In a powerful blender, mix the cashews, honey dates, and 1 cup of water until a thick cream develops. Slowly adding the remaining water, blend on high for 2 minutes. Strain the mixture through a nut milk bag, then gather the milk in a bowl.

6.62 ESSENTIAL NUT MILK

Ingredients:

1/2 cup raw almonds, shelled and soaked 2 cup liquid

1 banana, ripe, or 1 teaspoon maple syrup or honey (optional)

Instructions

Banana, honey, maple syrup, agave nectar, and one cup of water (if desired). Blend for an additional one to two minutes to get a cream that is smooth. While slowly adding the second cup of water to the blender, mix for 2 minutes. Place the strainer over a large basin and line it with cheesecloth or a cotton coffee filter. Pour the milk into the sieve gently and let it filter through, using a spatula to help the flow if required. A further half cup of nut milk can be obtained by rolling the cheesecloth's edges into a ball and then squeezing.

6.63 A FINE POT OF TEA

Ingredients:

4 tablespoons peppermint (dry)

12 teaspoons peppermint (fresh) 4 c. boiling water 1 tsp. honey (or more to taste)

Instructions

Add your herbs to a teapot once it has half-filled with hot water. Add water to the pot. To stop steam from leaving and carrying the taste and healing with it, cover the opening as soon as possible. Before filtering the tea into a cup via a fine-mesh tea strainer, let the herbs steep for 10 minutes. the honey is added for flavor.

6.64 SILKY CHAI (TEA) NUT MILK

Ingredients:

2 cups raw almonds, soaked (see Soaking Nuts and Seeds earlier in this chapter) 5 to 6 cups pure water

1 teaspoon vanilla extract

2 tablespoons raw honey or agave or 6 pitted dates (optional) 1 teaspoon nutmeg, or to taste

11 /2 teaspoon cinnamon, or to taste 1 /2 teaspoon cardamom, or to taste

Instructions:

Almonds that have been soaked in water should be added to a blender along with the liquid. Over a large mixing bowl, strain the mixture through a nut milk bag. Add the additional ingredients to the blender along with the milk, and mix just long enough to integrate everything.

6.65 LEMONADE

Ingredients:

6 lemons' juice (about 112 cups)

6 quarts of cold water 12 to 1 teaspoon stevia, or 1 cup Just Like Sugar

Instructions

In a large pitcher, mix the lemon juice, water, and sugar (or stevia) to taste. With a lemon slice or two for decoration, serve the lemonade over ice.

6.66 RICH AND MOIST CHOCOLATE CAKE

Ingredients:

½ cup brown rice flour

1/4 cup millet or sorghum flour 1/4 cup potato starch

1/4 cup tapioca flour 1/2 cup plus

2 tablespoons unsweetened cocoa powder 1 teaspoon xanthan gum

11/4 teaspoons baking soda 1 cup maple crystals

3/4 teaspoon sea salt

1 tablespoon organic vanilla 1/2 cup almond or rice milk

1 /2 cup Earth Balance margarine, room temperature, plus more for pan greasing 1 egg, beaten

3/4 cup brewed coffee, room temperature

Instructions

350 degrees Fahrenheit should be the oven's temperature setting. Margarine or coconut oil should be used to butter an 8-inch circular cake pan. You may also add and oil a circle of parchment paper if your pan has a tendency to cling. Combine the flours, potato starch, cocoa powder, xanthan

gum, baking soda, salt, and maple crystals in a large mixing basin. In a different, sizable mixing basin, combine the vanilla, milk, margarine, and egg using a hand mixer at a moderate speed. The dry ingredients should be added after you have started mixing with the hand mixer. Blend in the coffee well after that. The batter in the cake pan should have its top smoothed out. Bake for 30-35 minutes, flipping the pan halfway through, at 350°F in the oven. Transfer it from the oven when a toothpick inserted in the center comes out clean.

6.67 PINEAPPLE UPSIDE-DOWN CAKE

Ingredients:

2 cups almond flour, or more as needed for consistency 3 eggs, 4 tablespoons butter, melted 1/2 cup honey, 3/4 teaspoon organic vanilla extract 1/4 teaspoon cinnamon powder. 1 /2-pound fresh pineapple, thinly sliced (about 8 slices)

Instructions

350 degrees should be the prepared oven temperature. Grease a 9 by 12-inch baking dish with butter. Combine the almond flour, eggs, butter, honey, vanilla, and cinnamon until well-combined, either by hand or with a hand mixer. If necessary, add more almond flour to the mixture to prevent it from being too thin. Place the pineapple slices in a layer at the bottom of the baking dish. After uniformly spreading it out, pour the cake batter into the pan. 30–40 minutes of baking time, or until a toothpick inserted in the center of the cake comes out clean.

6.68 CHERRY COBBLER

Ingredients:

11/2 cups shredded coconut 11/2 cups walnuts

1/2 teaspoon salt 1/3 cup plus

1/2 cup pitted dates

3 cups frozen cherries, thawed and drained 2 teaspoons lemon juice

1/8 teaspoon cinnamon

Instructions

Combine the coconut, walnuts, and salt in a food processor. One at a time, until coarse crumbs form, process 1 1/3 cups pitted dates; put aside. Blend the remaining dates, cinnamon, lemon juice, and 1 cup of the cherries in a food processor. Blend the ingredients until it has chunks. In a large mixing basin, combine the remaining 2 cups of cherries. The cherry combination should fill a square glass baking dish halfway. Add crumble topping after placing in the refrigerator until ready to serve.

6.69 VEGAN LEMON MERINGUE PIE

Ingredients:

2 cups cashews, soaked Pinch of sea salt

4 tablespoons unsweetened coconut milk Juice of 1 lemon (about 1/4 cup)

2 to 4 tablespoons maple or agave syrup (optional)

4 to 8 tablespoons water

Lemon Meringue Pie Crust (see the following recipe) 1/4 cup unsweetened shredded coconut

Instructions

When the mixture resembles thick, creamy frosting, add the salt, coconut milk, cashews, lemon juice, syrup (if using), and half the water to a blender.Add the remaining water to the end to thin it down without causing the filling to separate. Sprinkle some shredded coconut on top after drizzling the mixture over the crust. Before cutting, place the pie in the refrigerator for 30 minutes to firm up.

6.70 LEMON MERINGUE PIE CRUST

Ingredients:

4 tablespoons ground flaxseed

4 tablespoons brown rice protein powder 1 /2 teaspoon stevia

1 to 2 teaspoons flaxseed oil 1 teaspoon cinnamon

1 teaspoon water

Instructions

The ground flaxseed, brown rice protein powder, stevia, flax seed oil, cinnamon, and water should all be combined in a 9-inch pie plate. The mixture should fill the pie plate's bottom.

6.71 BACON AND ZUCCHINI CRUSTLESS QUICHE

Ingredients

2 large zucchinis, grated

1½ cups (6 ounces/180 g) grated cheddar 2 tablespoons canola oil

6 large eggs, lightly beaten

Salt and freshly ground black pepper Green salad, for serving (optional)

Instructions

Turn the oven's temperature up to 350 degrees (170 degrees Celsius). Grease and line a 9-inch pie pan or quiche pan with parchment paper. Wrap a plate in paper towels. In a pan that is not yet hot, turn the heat to medium and add the bacon. Cook, tossing occasionally, for about ten minutes, or until crispy. Drain onto the ready-to-use plate. When the bacon has cooled enough to handle, shred it into small pieces.Combine the bacon, zucchini, cheese, oil, and eggs in a large mixing bowl. Pepper and salt to taste. In the baking dish, bake for 20 to 25 minutes, or until firm and golden brown. Removing from the oven and let stand for 5 minutes before slicing. If desired, serve it with a green salad on the side and warm or cooled.

6.72 SCRAMBLED EGGS

Ingredients

10 large eggs

¾ cup lactose-free milk

Salt and freshly ground black pepper 3 tablespoons salted butter

Toasted gluten-free, soy-free bread, for serving

Instructions

Crack the eggs into a large mixing basin, then whisk in the milk until thoroughly combined. Pepper and salt to taste. Melting the butter in a medium frying pan over low heat. In the pan, pour the egg mixture. Using a wooden spoon, gently press the egg mixture from the outer edges of the pan into the middle to prevent sticking. The eggs should continue to cook for a further 4 to 5 minutes, gently stirring once or twice, until almost done. The yolks should still be creamy and somewhat runny.

Serve immediately with toasted gluten-free bread.

6.73 OMELET WRAPS

Ingredients

Nonstick cooking spray 6 large eggs

6 thin slices cooked turkey breast

1 heaping tablespoon cranberry sauce

1 avocado, pitted, peeled, and sliced (optional) 1 tomato, sliced

2 handfuls of baby spinach leaves, rinsed and dried

1/2 cup (60 g) grated carrot (1 medium)

Instructions

Apply cooking spray to a medium nonstick frying pan and heat it to medium. One egg should be cracked and whisked with a fork in a small bowl. The omelet should be around 5 inches (12 cm) across when you pour the egg into the hot pan and tilt it to coat the bottom. Use a spatula or pancake-turner to flip the omelet, being cautious not to damage it, after cooking for 30 to 60 seconds. Remove it from the pan and arranging it on a dish after cooking for an additional 30 to 60 seconds. Repeat the process with the remaining eggs to make 6 omelets. Before serving, allow some cooling. To assemble, place an omelet on a flat surface. A piece of turkey breast, 1/2 teaspoon of cranberry sauce, some slices of avocado and tomato, some baby spinach leaves, and a sprinkle of carrot should all be placed in the center of the omelet. Fold the bottom third of the omelet toward the center, then the left and right edges to enclose the filling (almost as if you were rolling a burrito). Repeat the procedure with the remaining omelets and filling. Serve immediately or cover and chill until ready to eat.

6.74 LIGHT OMELET WITH CHICKEN AND SPINACH

Ingredients

4 large eggs, 1/4 cup roughly chopped basil

1/4 cup roughly chopped flat-leaf parsley Salt and freshly ground black pepper

1 tablespoon canola oil

1/2 cup shredded cooked chicken

A small handful of baby spinach leaves, rinsed, dried, and chopped 1/2 red bell pepper, diced

1/4 cup grated cheddar

Instructions

Eggs, basil, and parsley should all be whisked together in a medium mixing dish. Pepper and salt to taste. Temperature the oil in a medium frying pan over medium heat. Add the egg mixture, tilting the pan to coat the bottom as you do so. Cook till nearly set on top. With a spatula or pancake turner, gently lift the omelet's edges and shake it loose. Sprinkle the chicken, spinach, bell pepper, and cheese over one side of the omelet. Fold the second half over the filling to cover it. The mixture should be heated and the cheese should start to melt after a few minutes of cooking. Slice the omelet in half or serve it whole with two forks after removing it from the skillet. If preferred, divide the ingredients in half and make two smaller omelets.

6.75 ROASTED SWEET POTATO AND BELL PEPPER FRITTATA

Ingredients

1 large sweet potato, peeled (if desired) and chopped 2 red bell peppers, seeded and cut into quarters Olive oil for drizzling and greasing the pan

1 large handful of baby spinach leaves, rinsed and dried 10 large eggs

Salt and freshly ground black pepper

Instructions

Turn the oven's temperature up to 350 degrees (180 degrees Celsius). The sweet potato and bell peppers should be combined in a glass baking dish, drizzled with olive oil, and baked for 10 to 15 minutes, or until tender and golden brown. The pan should be taken out of the oven, covered with foil, and let to cool. Activate the oven. Cooled peppers should have their skins removed; discard them. Cut the peppers into substantial pieces using a broad knife. Grease a 9-inch (23-cm) oven-safe frying pan. The bottom layer is made of sweet potatoes, while the top layer is made of bell peppers. As a final touch, include a few spinach leaves. Bell peppers should be the last layer before moving on to the other vegetables. The eggs should be softly beaten and seasoned with salt and pepper in a bowl. In order to ensure that the eggs are well spread and cover any gaps, tilt the serving dish slightly as you pour the eggs over the vegetables. Cook for 20–30 minutes, or up to the center feels firm to the touch. The pan should be taken out of the oven and left to cool for five minutes before slicing.

6.76 CHEESE AND HERB SCONES

Ingredients

3/4 cup low-fat milk, lactose-free milk, or suitable plant-based milk, plus more for brushing

1 large egg

1/2 cup grated Parmesan 1/2 cup grated cheddar

3 to 4 heaping tablespoons chopped herbs (such as oregano, thyme, and flat-leaf parsley) 1 cup cornstarch, plus more for kneading

1 cup tapioca flour 1/2 cup soy flour

1 teaspoon xanthan gum or guar gum 2 teaspoons gluten-free baking powder

5 tablespoons unsalted butter, cut into cubes, at room temperature

Instructions

Turn the oven's temperature up to 400 degrees (200 degrees Celsius). A baking sheet should be lined with parchment paper. The milk and the egg should be combined in a mixing bowl. In a mixing dish, combine the Parmesan, cheddar, and herbs. Sift the cornstarch, tapioca flour, soy flour, xanthan gum, and baking powder three times in a medium mixing bowl (or whisk in the bowl until well combined). Rub the butter into the mixture using your hands until it resembles fine bread crumbs. Adding the milk mixture all at once and stir with a large metal spoon until the dough starts to come together. Dust your work surface lightly with cornstarch. Pulling the dough together gently with your hands, turn it out onto a floured surface. Pushing and turning the dough will help to softly knead it until it is just smooth (use a light touch, or the scones will be tough). Using a 2-inch (5-cm) biscuit or cookie cutter, cut out 10 to 12 scones from the dough after flattening it out to a thickness of 1 inch (2.5 cm) with a lightly floured rolling pin. Utilize a straight-down motion to do this (if you twist the cutter, the scones will rise unevenly during baking). Before each cut, dust the cutter with cornstarch to prevent sticking. The tops of the scones should be brushed with milk before being placed on the baking sheet at a distance of around 13 inches (1 cm). In the oven, bake for 10 to 12 minutes, or until well-done and golden brown. Cover the scones with a clean dish towel as soon as they come out of the oven (this will help give them a soft crust). Reheat the meal before serving.

6.77 CHOCOLATE SCONES

Ingredients

2/3 cup low-fat milk, lactose-free milk, or suitable plant-based milk, plus more for kneading

1 large egg

1 cup cornstarch, plus more for dusting 1 cup tapioca flour

1/2 cup soy flour

2 heaping tablespoons cocoa

1 teaspoon xanthan gum or guar gum 13/4 teaspoons gluten-free baking powder 1/4 cup superfine sugar

5 tablespoons unsalted butter, cut into cubes, at room temperature 1/2 cup chocolate chips*

Jam or butter, for serving

Instructions

Turn the oven's temperature up to 400 degrees (200 degrees Celsius). A baking sheet should be lined with parchment paper. The milk and the egg should be combined in a mixing bowl. Sift the cornstarch, tapioca flour, soy flour, cocoa, xanthan gum, baking powder, and sugar three times in a medium mixing bowl (or whisk in the bowl until well combined). Rub the butter into the mixture using your hands until it resembles fine bread crumbs. Stir the remaining Ingredients together before adding the chocolate chips. Add the milk and eggs all at once, mixing with a large metal spoon until the dough starts to come together. Dust your work surface lightly with cornstarch. Pulling the dough together gently with your hands, turn it out onto a floured surface. Pushing and turning the dough will help to softly knead it until it is just smooth (use a light touch, or the scones will be tough). Using a 2-inch (5-cm) biscuit or cookie cutter, cut out 10 to 12 scones from the dough after flattening it out to a thickness of 1 inch (2.5 cm) with a lightly floured rolling pin. Utilize a straight-down motion to do this (if you twist the cutter, the scones will rise unevenly during baking). Before each cut, dust the cutter with cornstarch to prevent sticking. Clean the tops of the scones with milk and arrange them on the baking sheet 13 inches (1 cm) apart. Cook for 10 to 12 minutes in the oven, or until well-done and golden brown. As soon as the scones are out of the oven, cover them with a fresh dish towel (this will help give them a soft crust). Butter and jam should be served warm.

6.78 BLUEBERRY PANCAKES

Ingredients

2 large eggs

1½ cups low-fat milk, lactose-free milk, or suitable plant-based milk 1 cup superfine white rice flour

½ cup (cornstarch ½ cup soy flour

2/3 cup packed light brown sugar

1 tablespoon plus 1 teaspoon gluten-free baking powder 1 teaspoon xanthan gum or guar gum

4 tablespoons salted butter, melted Nonstick cooking spray

1 cup fresh or frozen blueberries

Maple syrup and/or whipped cream, for serving (optional)

Instructions

In a little dish or liquid measuring cup, mix the milk and eggs together. Sift the rice flour, cornstarch, soy flour, brown sugar, baking powder, and xanthan gum three times in a large mixing basin (or whisk in the bowl until well combined). Create a well in the middle, then gently pour the milk mixture in while whisking everything together. Add the melted butter and then set aside for 15 minutes. Cooking spray a sizable nonstick frying pan or griddle, then heat it on medium.Pour roughly 1/2 cup/125 ml of batter each pancake, in batches, to form four 4-inch (10-cm) pancakes, and cook them for one minute, or until they start to firm up. After each pancake is topped with 8 blueberries, cook for an additional 2 minutes. To ensure thorough cooking, cook for a further 2 minutes. Transfer to a plate and covering loosely with foil to keep warm. Repeat the process with the remaining batter and berries to make a total of 12 pancakes. For an extra delightful treat, serve right away with any remaining blueberries, maple syrup (if desired), and/or whipped cream.

6.79 PUMPKIN MUFFINS

Ingredients

1 cup superfine white rice flour ½ cup cornstarch
½ cup potato flour

2 teaspoons gluten-free baking powder 1 teaspoon baking soda

1 teaspoon xanthan gum or guar gum 2 teaspoons pumpkin pie spice

1 heaping tablespoon ground cinnamon 3 tablespoons unsalted butter, melted

3⁄4 cup (200 g) gluten-free, low-fat vanilla yogurt 2 large eggs

11⁄2 cups mashed cooked pumpkin, kabocha, or other suitable winter squash (from about 18

500 g peeled and seeded raw squash) 1 cup superfine sugar

Instructions

To make a 12-cup muffin tray, preheat the oven to 325 degrees Fahrenheit (170 degrees Celsius) and line the cups with paper liners. Sift the rice flour, cornstarch, potato flour, baking soda, xanthan gum, pumpkin pie spice, and cinnamon three times in a large mixing basin (or whisk in the bowl until well combined). Combine the melted butter, yogurt, and eggs in a medium mixing bowl. In a mixing dish, combine the squash and sugar. With a heavy metal spoon, add to the flour mixture and stir until just combined (do not overmix). the batter into the muffin cups until they are two-thirds full. Bake for 15-20 minutes, or until toothpick inserted in the middle of the cake comes out clean and the top is golden brown. Cool in the pan for five minutes before transferring to a wire rack to finish cooling.

6.80 BANANA–CHOCOLATE CHIP MUFFINS

Ingredients

1 cup superfine white rice flour ½ cup cornstarch ½ cup soy flour

2 teaspoons gluten-free baking powder 1 teaspoon baking soda

1 teaspoon xanthan gum or guar gum 2 large eggs

1 cup superfine sugar

3 tablespoons unsalted butter, melted 1 teaspoon vanilla extract

2 bananas, peeled and mashed

⅓ cup low-fat milk, lactose-free milk, or suitable plant-based milk ¾ cup gluten-free, low-fat vanilla yogurt

1 cup chocolate chips

Instructions

To make a 12-cup muffin tray, preheat the oven to 325 degrees Fahrenheit (170 degrees Celsius) and line the cups with paper liners. Sift the rice flour, cornstarch, soy flour, baking powder, baking soda, and xanthan gum three times in a large mixing basin (or whisk in the bowl until well combined). The eggs and sugar should be whisked together in a medium mixing basin until foamy and thick. Add the melted butter, vanilla, mashed bananas, milk, and yogurt to a large mixing bowl (do not overmix). Add to the flour mixture and beat with a heavy metal spoon until just combined. The chocolate bits are carefully folded in. the batter into the muffin cups until they are two-thirds full. Up to a toothpick placed in the center of the cake comes out clean, bake for 15 to 20 minutes.

6.81 VANILLA-RHUBARB MUFFINS

Ingredients

1¼ cup finely chopped rhubarb 1½ cups superfine sugar

1 cup superfine white rice flour ½ cup tapioca flour ½ cup cornstarch

2 teaspoons gluten-free baking powder 1 teaspoon baking soda

1 teaspoon xanthan gum or guar gum 3 tablespoons unsalted butter, melted ½ teaspoon vanilla extract

¾ cup gluten-free, low-fat vanilla yogurt

2 large eggs

Instructions

The rhubarb should be combined with 14 cups (55 g) of sugar and covered in water in a small pot. High heat is used to bring to a boil, then medium heat is used to simmer the food for 10 minutes, or until the veggies are tender. Remove the water and leave it to cool. To make a 12-cup muffin tray, preheat the oven to 325 degrees Fahrenheit (170 degrees Celsius) and line the cups with paper liners. Sift the rice flour, tapioca flour, cornstarch, baking powder, baking soda, and xanthan gum three times in a large mixing basin (or whisk in the bowl until well combined). Melted butter, vanilla, yogurt, eggs, and the remaining 114 cups (275 g) sugar should be combined in a medium mixing bowl. The yogurt mixture should be gently incorporated into the flour mixture using a large metal spoon. The ingredients shouldn't be overmixed. Add the cooked rhubarb and gently stir (take care because you want the pieces to remain intact). Two-thirds of the way up the muffin cups should be filled with batter. 12 to 15 minutes in the oven, or until the muffins are golden brown and a toothpick stuck in the cente comes out clean.r Cool for five minutes in the pan before moving to a wire rack to cool the rest of the way.

6.82 GINGER AND PECAN MUFFINS

Ingredients

1 cup superfine white rice flour 1/2 cup tapioca flour 1/2 cup cornstarch

2 teaspoons gluten-free baking powder 1 teaspoon baking soda

1 teaspoon xanthan gum or guar gum 3 tablespoons unsalted butter, melted

3/4 cup gluten-free, low-fat vanilla yogurt 2 large eggs

1¼ cups superfine sugar

½ cup roughly chopped pecans

½ cup chopped crystallized ginger, plus 12 small pieces for garnish

Instructions

To make a 12-cup muffin tray, preheat the oven to 325 degrees Fahrenheit (170 degrees Celsius) and line the cups with paper liners. Sift the rice flour, tapioca flour, cornstarch, baking powder, baking soda, and xanthan gum three times in a large mixing basin (or whisk in the bowl until well combined). Combine the melted butter, yogurt, eggs, sugar, pecans, and ginger in a medium mixing dish. With a heavy metal spoon, add to the flour mixture and stir until just combined. (Avoid overmixing.Before baking, top the batter with a piece of crystallized ginger that is about two-thirds full. Bake the cake for 15 to 20 minutes, or until the top is golden brown and a toothpick inserted in the center of the cake comes out clean. Cool in the pan for five minutes before transferring to a wire rack to finish cooling.

6.83 CHEESY CORN MUFFINS

Ingredients

1 cup superfine white rice flour ½ cup cornstarch

½ cup tapioca flour

2 teaspoons gluten-free baking powder 1 teaspoon baking soda

1 teaspoon xanthan gum or guar gum 3 tablespoons salted butter, melted

¾ cup gluten-free, low-fat plain yogurt 3 large eggs

½ cup grated cheddar, plus twelve ⅓-inch cubes ½ cup finely grated Parmesan

4 to 6 lean bacon slices, cooked until crispy and crumbled (optional) 1 cup drained canned or thawed frozen corn kernels

Pinch of salt and freshly ground black pepper

Instructions

To make a 12-cup muffin tray, preheat the oven to 325 degrees Fahrenheit (170 degrees Celsius) and line the cups with paper liners. Sift the rice flour, cornstarch, tapioca flour, baking powder, baking soda, and xanthan gum three times in a large mixing basin (or whisk in the bowl until well combined). Melted butter, yogurt, eggs, cheddar, Parmesan, bacon (if using), and corn should all be combined in a medium mixing bowl. With a large metal spoon, stir the yogurt mixture into the flour mixture until everything is thoroughly combined (do not overmix). Pepper and salt to taste. Halfway fill the muffin cups with batter, then top each with a cheddar cheese cube. With the remaining batter, fill the cups two thirds of the way. A toothpick put into the center of a muffin (but avoiding the cheese filling) should come out clean after baking for 15 to 20 minutes. Cool in the pan for five minutes before transferring to a wire rack to finish cooling.

6.84 SPINACH AND TOMATO MUFFINS

Ingredients

1 cup superfine white rice flour ½ cup cornstarch

½ cup soy flour

2 teaspoons gluten-free baking powder 1 teaspoon baking soda

1 teaspoon xanthan gum or guar gum 5 tablespoons salted butter, melted

¾ cup gluten-free, low-fat plain yogurt 3 large eggs

1 cup low-fat milk, lactose-free milk, or suitable plant-based milk 1 cup finely grated Parmesan

2 medium tomatoes, diced

2 ounces baby spinach leaves, rinsed, dried, and roughly chopped Pinch of salt and freshly ground black pepper

Instructions

A 12-cup muffin tray should be lined with paper liners. Set the oven's temperature to 325°F (170°C). To make a big bowl, three times sift the rice flour, cornstarch, soy flour, baking powder, baking soda, and xanthan gum (or whisk in the bowl until well combined). In a medium bowl, mix the melted butter, yogurt, eggs, milk, Parmesan, tomatoes, spinach, salt, and pepper. With a wooden spoon, stir the addition with the flour mixture until barely incorporated. When the muffin cups are two-thirds filled, evenly distribute the batter into each one. A toothpick put into the center of a muffin should come out clean after baking for 15 to 20 minutes, or up to the muffins are firm to the touch. After 5 minutes, remove from the pan and let cool fully on a wire rack.

6.85 HIGH-FIBER MUFFINS WITH ZUCCHINI AND SUNFLOWER SEEDS

Ingredients

1 cup brown rice flour 1/2 cup cornstarch

1/2 cup soy flour

2 teaspoons gluten-free baking powder 1 teaspoon baking soda

1 teaspoon xanthan gum or guar gum 5 tablespoons salted butter, melted

1/2 cup low-fat milk, lactose-free milk, or suitable plant-based milk 3/4 cup gluten-free, low-fat plain yogurt

3 large eggs

¾ cup (60 g) finely grated Parmesan ½ medium zucchini, grated

½ cup (75 g) roasted unsalted sunflower seeds ½ cup (60 g) rice bran

¼ cup (25 g) walnuts, crushed

¼ teaspoon freshly grated nutmeg

Pinch of salt and freshly ground black pepper

Instructions

A 12-cup muffin tray should be lined with paper liners. Set the oven's temperature to 325°F (170°C). To make a big bowl, three times sift the rice flour, cornstarch, soy flour, baking powder, baking soda, and xanthan gum (or whisk in the bowl until well combined). In a medium bowl, stir together the melted butter, milk, yogurt, eggs, Parmesan, zucchini, sunflower seeds, rice bran, walnuts, nutmeg, salt, and pepper. Add the flour mixture and stir for two to three minutes with a wooden spoon (be careful not to overmix). When the muffin cups are two-thirds filled, evenly distribute the batter into each one. A toothpick put into the center of a muffin should come out clean after baking for 15 - 20 minutes, or until the muffins are firm to the touch. After 5 minutes, remove from the pan and let cool fully on a wire rack.

6.86 CHILI-CHEESE MUFFINS

Ingredients

1 cup superfine white rice flour ½ cup cornstarch

½ cup soy flour

2 teaspoons gluten-free baking powder 1 teaspoon baking soda

1 teaspoon xanthan gum or guar gum 1 teaspoon chili powder

5 tablespoons salted butter, melted

¾ cup gluten-free, low-fat plain yogurt 3 large eggs

¾ cup low-fat milk, lactose-free milk, or suitable plant-based milk ¾ cup finely grated Parmesan

1 cup grated cheddar

2 heaping tablespoons finely chopped flat-leaf parsley Pinch of salt and freshly ground black pepper

Instructions

To make a 12-cup muffin tray, preheat the oven to 325 degrees Fahrenheit (170 degrees Celsius) and line the cups with paper liners. Sift the rice flour, cornstarch, soy flour, baking soda, xanthan gum, and chili powder together three times in a large mixing basin (or whisk in the bowl until well combined). Melted butter, yogurt, eggs, milk, Parmesan, cheddar, parsley, salt, and pepper should all be combined in a medium mixing basin. Add to the flour mixture and beat with a heavy metal spoon until just combined. Put about half a cup of batter in each muffin cup. The muffins are done when they feel firm when touched and a toothpick put into the center comes out clean, usually after about 20 minutes in the oven. Set aside for five minutes to cool in the pan before transferring to a wire rack to cool completely.

6.87 SMOOTHIE MAGIC

Ingredients

Half cup Strawberries

1 cup milk(Lactogen free) Frozen cubes

Instructions

To get a smooth mixture, blend all the ingredients together.

6.88 GOLDEN FRENCH TOAST

Ingredients

4 large eggs

½ cup lactose-free milk

1 teaspoon vanilla extract

8 ounces sourdough bread or low-FODMAP gluten-free bread 1 teaspoon ground cinnamon

1 tablespoon butter, or more if needed

Instructions

Combining eggs, milk, and vanilla extract in a 9x13-inch baking dish and stir together. Soak the bread in the mixture of eggs and milk. Use a lot of cinnamon. Sprinkled. In a large, well-seasoned cast-iron frying pan or nonstick skillet, melt a teaspoon of butter over medium heat. Once the butter is boiling, add the bread pieces in a single layer to the pan. Wait until the bottoms of the bread are golden brown, about 2 to 3 minutes. You should flip it over while cooking to get a golden brown color on the opposite side. The toasts are made when they have a small dome in the center. Use the leftover bread and butter (2 tablespoons) to make another sandwich. The French toast can be served immediately or kept warm on a baking sheet in an oven preheated to 200 degrees Fahrenheit.

6.89 HUMMINGBIRD MUFFINS

Ingredients

1 large egg

¼ cup packed light brown sugar ¼ cup neutral-flavored oil

¼ cup crushed pineapple, drained ¾ cup mashed ripe banana

¾ cup mashed ripe banana 1 tablespoon chia seeds

¼ cup/25g sorghum flour

½ cup/55g Authentic Foods Superfine Brown Rice Flour 2 tablespoons tapioca starch

1 tablespoon cornstarch

1 tablespoon arrowroot powder 2 teaspoons baking powder

¼ teaspoon salt

1 teaspoon ground cinnamon ¼ cup chopped walnuts Cooking spray

1 tablespoon coarse sugar crystals

Instructions

To make the batter, whisk together the egg, brown sugar, oil, pineapple, and banana in a large bowl. To incorporate the chia seeds, stir them into the egg mixture. Dough should be thick enough to be spooned after being mixed with sorghum flour, rice flour, tapioca starch, cornstarch, arrowroot powder, baking powder, salt, and cinnamon. Incorporate the walnuts and stir to combine. The batter has to rest for 15 minutes. Bake at 350 degrees Fahrenheit. Prepare a muffin tin that holds six cups by spraying it with cooking spray. Before dividing the mixture among the muffin cups, give the batter one more stir. Each muffin should be dusted with sugar. Baking for 25 to 30 minutes at 350 degrees

Fahrenheit, or up to firm. Allow it cool in the pan for a few minutes, then transfer to a cooling rack to finish cooling. You may eat it right away, store it in the fridge for up to a day, or even freeze it for up to six months.months if stored in an airtight container.

6.90 SWEET POTATO HASH

Ingredients

1 medium sweet potato (¾ pound)

2 tablespoons garlic-infused olive oil 1 small onion, sliced

1 small summer squash (about ¾ pound), diced 10 medium radishes (about ½ pound), chopped ½ cup chopped scallion greens

Instructions

Once the sweet potato has been pierced multiple times, microwave it for 4 to 6 minutes on high, or until it can be easily pierced. Slice the unpeeled sweet potato into bite-sized pieces after it is cool enough to handle. In a broad skillet over medium heat, warm the oil. The onion is added and sautéed until transparent. Remove and discard. In a pan, sauté the squash and radishes for three minutes. While stirring occasionally, let the sweet potato brown on the bottom for 8 to 10 minutes. With a spatula, remove the vegetable mixture from the pan's bottom, turn it gently, and cook for an additional 5 minutes. Garnish with scallion greens and serve right away.

6.91 BREAKFAST SCONES

Ingredients:

2 cups (300 g) cornstarch

2 cups (250 g) tapioca flour 1 cup (90 g) soy flour

2 teaspoons xanthan gum

1 tablespoon baking powder (gluten-free if following a gluten-free diet) ½ cup superfine sugar 10 tablespoons unsalted butter, at room temperature, cut into cubes 1 ¼ cups low-fat milk, plus 2 tablespoons (preferably cow's milk) 2 eggs

Jam, optional

Whipped cream, optional

Instructions:

Turn the oven's temperature up to 400 degrees (200 degrees Celsius). Cornstarch should be used to dust and oil a baking sheet. Sift the cornstarch, tapioca flour, soy flour, xanthan gum, baking powder, and sugar three times in a large mixing basin (or mix with a whisk to ensure they are well combined). The mixture should resemble fine bread crumbs after you've added the butter and kept cutting. 1 cup of milk and the eggs should be whisked together in a mixing bowl. Stir into the flour mixture as soon as the dough starts to come together.Pulling the dough together gently with your hands, turn it out onto a surface that has been lightly dusted with flour. The dough should be smooth after four or five repetitions of kneading. The dough should be rolled out to a 1 inch thickness (3 cm). To cut out the scones, use a 2-inch (5-cm) biscuit or cookie cutter. When using the cutter, move it straight downward; if you twist it, the scones will rise unevenly. Cornstarch applied on the cutter before each cut is also beneficial. On the baking sheet, space the scones 12 inches (or 1 centimeter) apart. The leftover milk should be brushed on top. Bake until golden and cooked through for 15 to 18 minutes, rotating the sheet halfway through. The moment the scones are taken out of the oven, cover them with a fresh kitchen towel (this gives them a soft crust). After 5 minutes, top the scones with jam and whipped cream, if you'd like.

6.92 HAND-MILLED BREAKFAST CEREAL   GLUTEN-FREE

Ingredients:

1/4 cup long-grain brown rice 1/4 cup millet

1/4 cup quinoa (red or white)

1/4 cup walnut or other nut pieces, ground if nut pieces are irritating 1/4 cup dried blueberries

1/2 teaspoon cinnamon Pinch of salt

11/2 cups water

1/4 cup organic whole milk or non-dairy milk (such as unsweetened Rice Dream) Grade B maple syrup (optional)

Butter or coconut oil (optional)

Instructions:

Grind the quinoa, millet, and rice in a powerful blender or a coffee/spice grinder. In a mixing dish, combine the ground grains, nuts, and blueberries that have been dried, cinnamon, salt, and water. Bring to a boil, then abate heat to low. Stir often and simmer for 10 to 15 minutes, covering the pan, if needed, to get the appropriate consistency. Add the milk, syrup, and butter as desired.

6.93 CARAMELIZED BANANA AND DATE "PORRIDGE" (SCD)

Ingredients:

1 banana 2 dates

1 teaspoon butter

1/2 a head of cauliflower, pureed Dash of cinnamon

1/2 to 1 tablespoon honey (optional)

Instructions:

Bananas should be cut into wedges. Pit the dates, then cut them into little pieces. Melt the butter over a medium-high heat in a small frying pan. Add the banana and dates to the melted butter and stir constantly for the next two to three minutes. Once the banana starts to turn brown, drop the heat to medium and add the pureed cauliflower. Heat to a very high degree. If desired, top with honey and sprinkle cinnamon on top of it.

6.94 SOAKED OATS PORRIDGE

Ingredients:

2 cups organic oat groats 1/4 cup dried figs

1 tablespoon walnuts

1 tablespoon shredded coconut

1 cup coconut juice or water to mix ingredients

4 ounces of coconut milk Pinch of cinnamon or nutmeg (optional)

Instructions:

The previous evening, combine the oats, figs, almonds, and coconut shreds in a dish and cover with water to soak overnight. To get rid of any leftovers, properly rinse the components in new water in the morning. In a blender or food processor, combining the soaking mixture with the coconut juice or water and process until smooth. Before serving, pour the coconut milk over the other ingredients and season with a little cinnamon or nutmeg (if desired).

6.95 STRAWBERRIES AND CREAM OATMEAL

Ingredients:

1 cup quick-cooking rolled oats 2 cups water

1 banana, cut up

5 strawberries, cut up 2 ounces coconut milk

Instructions:

The rolled oats and water should be combined on a cold burner. Bring to a boil, then turn the heat down to low and simmer for an additional five minutes. Combine the banana and strawberries in a mixing dish, then add the oats and coconut milk.

6.96 CINNAMON PANCAKES WITH GHEE

Ingredients:

1 cup whole organic cashews 1 /2 teaspoon baking soda

3 eggs

1 tablespoon Kendall's SCD Dairy Yogurt Splash of vanilla

Pinch of salt

2 tablespoons of honey 1 teaspoon cinnamon

1 tablespoon coconut oil

Instructions:

Using a food processor, make a paste out of the cashews. The baking soda, eggs, yogurt, vanilla, salt, honey, and cinnamon should all be combined.

Coconut oil should be melted in a frying pan over low heat in the oven. Pour the batter into the pan in 14-cup batches. Flip when it's golden.

6.97 GRATIFYING GHEE

Ingredients:

1 pound unsalted butter

Instructions:

Melt the butter gradually over low heat in a big pot with a thick bottom. Stirring is prohibited. Cook the butter at a low temperature until it has melted and transformed into a transparent, golden liquid. It won't boil over if you have a deep enough pot since it will bubble and foam. The milk solids may settle to the bottom of the pan and turn golden or light brown in color. It is possible to skim off and remove the dense foam. When the liquid has reached a clear gold hue, turn off the heat. The color of overdone ghee is darker. Set the sieve over a clean saucepan with the four sheets of cheesecloth inside. The still-hot ghee should be strained using the sieve. Put the strained ghee in a tidy container with a secure lid.

6.98 GLUTEN-FREE PUMPKIN SPICE BREAD

Ingredients:

3 large eggs 2 cups sugar

1/2 cup grapeseed oil

One 15-ounce can of organic pumpkin 2 teaspoons vanilla

2 cups gluten-free flour

11 /2 teaspoons xanthan gum 1 teaspoon baking powder

1 teaspoon baking soda 2 teaspoons cinnamon

1/2 teaspoon ground cloves 3/4 teaspoon nutmeg

3/4 teaspoon ground ginger 1 teaspoon sea salt

Instructions:

350 degrees Fahrenheit should be the oven's temperature setting. Set aside two loaf pans that have been lined with parchment paper and coated with olive oil. Use a hand mixer to whip the eggs in a medium mixing bowl until frothy. The sugar should be beaten in until the mixture is entirely smooth. With a spatula, fold in the oil, pumpkin, and vanilla essence. In a another bowl, combine the remaining ingredients. In a mixing basin, combine the dry and wet ingredients and whisk well. Bake the mixture for 35 minutes, flipping the pans over halfway through. Pour the mixture into the prepared pans. When a toothpick or wooden skewer placed into the center of the loaf comes out clean, the bread is finished baking. Place a cooling wire rack underneath.

6.99 BANANA BREAD

Ingredients:

2 cups finely ground almond flour 1 /2 teaspoon baking soda

1/2 teaspoon salt 1/4 cup honey

1 large ripe banana, mashed 3 large eggs

Instructions:

Grease a 9-by-5-inch loaf pan and line it with parchment paper before preheating the oven to 300 degrees. Almond flour, baking soda, and salt should all be combined in a mixing bowl. Eggs, honey, and mashed banana are well combined. After adding the liquid components, mix the dry ingredients together until well-combined. Bake the loaf for 40 minutes, or until a knife inserted in the center comes out clean. Pour the mixture into the prepared loaf pan. Permit cooling.

7   CONCLUSION

Crohn's is unpredictable, and each person's experience with Crohn's disease is different. Some people rarely experience flare-ups, while others experience them frequently. If you are prone to flares or are currently undergoing one, remember that you're not alone. Almost everyone with Crohn's will encounter a flare-up at some point.

There isn't one diet that works for everyone with inflammatory bowel disease, including Crohn's. Many people with the condition use elements of low-fiber, low-fat, and low-FODMAP diets to create a plan that helps them manage Crohn's. During times when they are having symptom flares, it can be useful to stick to a BRAT diet, though this is only a temporary measure. If you have Crohn's, you may find it helpful to work with a registered dietician or nutritionist to design a Crohn's diet plan that suits your unique dietary needs and tastes.